Recalled by Life

Recalled by Life

Anthony J. Sattilaro, M.D.
with Tom Monte

Boston
HOUGHTON MIFFLIN COMPANY

Library of Congress Cataloging in Publication Data

Sattilaro, Anthony J.
Recalled by life.

1. Sattilaro, Anthony J.   2. Cancer—Patients—
United States—Biography.   3. Cancer—Diet therapy.
4. Prostate gland—Cancer—Patients—United States—
Biography.   I. Monte, Tom.
RC265.6.S27A37   1982   362.1'96994'00924 [B]   82-6077
ISBN 0-395-32524-2

S 10 9 8 7 6 5

To the Lamb of God,
Who takes away the Sin of the World
and Grants Us Peace.

For what shall it profit a man,
if he shall gain the whole world,
and lose his own soul?

MARK 8:36

Foreword

*T*HIS BOOK concerns the period of my life from May 1978 to the summer of 1981. During that time, I encountered many ideas that the reader will doubtless find foreign and, perhaps, even disturbing. Certainly, that was my initial reaction. My hope is that the reader will keep an open mind.

I offer this book as a message of hope and as an attempt to stimulate new ideas in the prevention and treatment of serious illness, particularly cancer. However, there is no magic bullet to be found in these pages, no remedy for malignancy such as that provided by penicillin in the fight against infectious disease. This is the story of one man's experience in a long process toward regaining his health, a process that involved many factors. Among the most important of these were dramatic changes in diet and lifestyle, as well as a sustaining faith that all things are possible with the help of the Creator. No one aspect of this process can be taken as the sole reason for my change in health. Rather, the reader should recognize that my recovery was the result of a totality of many factors, which have yet to be shown as reproducible in others.

Until scientific evidence demonstrates that diet plays a significant role in the treatment of cancer—or any other illness, for that matter—I cannot endorse any regimen as a replacement for standard Western medical treatment.

Finally, and most importantly, I urge every reader to consult his or her own physician before making any dramatic change in diet, particularly the one discussed in this book. This is especially important if one has already been diagnosed as having a serious illness and would like to use diet as a complement to traditional therapy. Unless one consults a physician or a trained nutritionist, major alterations in diet can result in harmful side effects.

My story is not meant to serve the interests of any single group or so-called movement. My hope is that the ideas presented here will be tested under scientifically controlled conditions and that such studies will give rise to a new and more effective means of health care. To that end I offer my story.

ANTHONY J. SATTILARO, M.D.

Recalled by Life

Chapter 1

IN JUNE 1978, I was told by my physicians that I had cancer. The medical diagnosis was that I had prostatic cancer, stage IV (D), which had metastasized to other parts of my body, including my skull, shoulder, spine, sternum, and ribs. I was forty-seven years old. My doctors informed me that I had perhaps "a few" years to live, and I knew those years would be spent in a torturous slide toward death. I was already suffering from acute back pain, for which large doses of painkiller provided only periodic relief.

Within weeks after the diagnosis was made, I underwent surgery and began estrogen treatment to combat the spread of the disease. It soon became apparent, however, that this would not halt the malignancy, and in light of this I began to seek alternatives that might rescue me from death. I had been a doctor for more than twenty years by then, and it was with no small trepidation that I went looking for answers outside the profession to which I had dedicated my life. This search put me on an extraordinary journey — one that has led me not only to a restoration of my health, but to the very roots of my being.

In light of the seriousness of my disease and the fact that

cancer has proved in most cases to be intractable to current methods of treatment, I believe my story could be of benefit to others. Public opinion polls show that cancer is the most feared disease in America. Approximately 700,000 people in the United States will contract cancer this year alone, and nearly half a million will die of it. It is the second leading killer disease in the nation, trailing only cardiovascular disease in the number of dead it leaves in its wake. As yet, there is no cure for cancer. Certain therapeutic measures, such as surgery, chemotherapy, radiation, and x-rays — in some instances — have been shown to control the disease and prolong life. In most cases, however, cancer is unstoppable. The chances of anyone defeating the disease once they have been afflicted are about one in three, the same ratio that existed in 1950. More people will contract cancer this year than in any other year of this nation's history; nevertheless, that number will be surpassed by 1983, and surpassed again by 1984 if better preventive measures are not taken.

Anecdotal evidence, such as my own story, is not regarded as scientific proof of anything. Yet, as a physician who has experienced firsthand the trauma of cancer, I feel it of the highest importance to report my case history in the hope that it may stimulate scientific research and, perhaps, new ideas that may eventually lead to a more effective treatment — if not a cure — for this dread disease.

My story begins on May 23, 1978, a cool, overcast day in Philadelphia, Pennsylvania. That Tuesday morning I awoke with the same dull back pain that had been with me for the previous two years. I had been in the routine of waking up and going straight into the bathroom, swallowing a couple of painkillers — the first of many needed to get me through the day — and chasing them down with some water. I would then get into the shower and let the hot water pound the back pain into remission. This morning was no different from any other, except that I was aware that the back pain seemed a bit more intense than usual.

After the shower, I shaved and dressed. Just before I left for the office, I combed my hair before the mirror and took a long look at my face. My dark brown hair was becoming increasingly gray. My face was fleshy and pale. My brown eyes had lost their brightness many years ago, but now the irises were yellow-brown and bloodshot. Below my eyes were two large and swollen bags of puffy skin. Two long and deep lines ran from the corners of my nose to the corners of my mouth and then down to my chin. At 150 pounds, my five-foot-five-inch frame was only a few pounds overweight, but I felt loose and flabby. This was the main reason I had begun riding my bicycle to and from work each day. The signs of old age were setting in, and I wanted to hold them off for as long as possible. Looking into the mirror now, I could see that it was going to take more than a couple of bicycle rides each day to recover any of my lost youth. I got the bicycle out of the closet and headed for the elevator.

I live on the twenty-seventh floor of a cooperative apartment complex in the heart of Philadelphia, near Rittenhouse Square. Fancy Square, as it is called by the locals, is a small patch of green amid Philadelphia's inner city affluence. The square is crowned with a large fountain; surrounding the square are some of the most elegant and expensive apartments and condominiums in the city. I rode my bicycle to the Union League, a men's club I belong to, where I ate breakfast. After breakfast I continued on to my office at Methodist Hospital in South Philadelphia.

I rode along the right side of 15th Street. The bleak, gray sky somehow made the tall buildings on either side of me seem looming and ominous. Traffic was heavy. As I approached the intersection of 15th and Washington streets, a man suddenly darted in front of me from the sidewalk. I swerved to my left to avoid him, barely missed being hit by a car, and saw too late the gaping jaws of a large pothole. The bike shuddered as the front wheel dropped into the crater. The world spun around, and I went down hard. The palms of my hands and groin took the full impact of the fall. As I lay in the street near the curb, people hurried around me. Fortunately, I was out of the way of traffic. I got up and dusted myself off, cursing out loud as I pulled a few imbedded asphalt pebbles from the skin of my palms. My right testicle was screaming with pain. After a few minutes, I collected myself, got back on the bike, and painfully rode to my office.

I arrived at my office with my back and testicle pulsating with pain. I immediately telephoned my internist and made an appointment for the following week. I then painfully settled back into my chair, took an electric heating pad from my desk drawer, and placed it behind my back. I popped a couple more analgesics into my mouth and turned my attention to the mound of paperwork and little pink telephone messages that stared up at me from the desk.

Once the painkillers took effect, I had little trouble putting my own health problems out of my mind and concentrating on my job. There was much to do. Six months before this spring day, I had been appointed chief executive officer of Methodist Hospital. Methodist is an old institution, dating back nearly a hundred years. It is now a modern hospital, with just over two hundred and fifty beds and about eleven hundred employees. Hospital administration was a new career for me. I had been a member of the hospital's medical staff for the past thirteen years, serving as an anesthesiologist. In December 1977 I was appointed to my newest position.

Now I was facing my first real test: a major inspection of the hospital's facilities, policies, and staff by the Pennsylvania Department of Health. The inspection would review every facet of the hospital's operation: our surgical procedures, our treatment of various illnesses, the condition and maintenance of our equipment in every department, the state of our acute care wards and emergency rooms, the cleanliness of the hospital, the efficiency of our administration, and the food in our cafeteria. The inspection would take place during the first week in June. Then the Department of Health would determine whether Methodist should be reissued its license to provide health care. Every hospital in the country goes through several inspections each year, and this was one of the most important for us. As chief executive officer, my job was to see that the hospital was running at the peak of efficiency and that all departments were providing the very best service possible. We were now in the process of taking care of last-minute details; each day I made my way through the wards, conducting my own inspection of the facilities and staff.

During my years at Methodist, I had been through these inspections many times, but this one was different. My appointment as chief executive officer had been a controversial one, and it prompted a couple of people to resign from the staff in protest. The argument was that I had had little experience as a hospital administrator and that there were other, more qualified candidates to choose from. On top of this was the standing rationale that physicians make poor administrators. Still, I was not without my strong points as a candidate for the post. I had been chairman of the department of anesthesiology for several years. I had also studied hospital administration at Harvard University's Business School and School of Public Health. My training at Harvard was geared toward filling the role of chief executive officer of a health care institution. Further, my experience at Methodist had given me an insider's view of the problems of the institution and how best to handle them.

Although the hospital's Board of Trustees offered me the job, they demonstrated their own apprehensions by refusing to change my contract from chairman of anesthesiology to hospital administrator. This was a clear statement by the board; I was, in effect, on probation. Thus, I viewed the upcoming inspection with some trepidation, realizing that it was as much an assessment of my own performance as it was an examination of the hospital. I realized, too, that the inspection team's judgment would be reflected dramatically in my future at Methodist. A less than enthusiastic report from the Department of Health might well send me back to anesthesia, but a complimentary assessment would solidify my position.

Despite some anxiety over the arrival of the inspection team, I was confident of my own skills and the condition of the hospital. I had quickly come to feel confident in my new post, and I knew I could run the institution better than any of my peers. In fact, I looked forward to receiving the health inspectors.

Apart from falling off my bicycle and my increasingly painful back, May 23 was a routine day. That night I had dinner with H. Robert Cathcart, president of the Pennsylvania Hospital. We dined at Bookbinder's restaurant, seated under the smiling eyes of so many celebrities, whose framed photographs hang on the walls.

It was my custom to eat all my meals in restaurants. I have never been married and learned early in my adult life to detest the kitchen. I thought myself fortunate that I could afford this luxury, but, considering my antipathy for cooking, there seemed no other way short of hiring a cook. Eating at a restaurant seemed simpler. Like most affluent Americans, I ate meat at nearly every meal, from bacon and sausage in the morning to steak and prime rib at night. I rarely ate fish, and when I did I considered it a break from the norm. That evening, I ordered my usual V.O. to start the meal; the entrée was prime rib, with baked potato and sour cream, vegetables glazed in butter, and, later, a large dessert. I enjoyed dessert more than any other part of the meal, and I sometimes treated myself to two if I felt my weight was sufficiently under control at the time. The key issue with food was keeping my weight down.

Bob Cathcart and I talked at length about the inspection Methodist would be undergoing. Bob had been president of Pennsylvania Hospital for some time, and I often looked to him for advice. After a time, the conversation shifted to more personal matters and eventually he asked me about my father.

For a moment, I thought about my father and all that he had been through during the previous six months. In November 1977, physicians at Jefferson Hospital in Philadelphia had removed a malignant tumor from his right lung. My father's surgeon, Dr. John Templeton, a friend of mine, told me that he believed he had gotten the entire tumor, but it was impossible to say for sure since part of it could have gotten into the blood stream and spread to other areas of the body. In the weeks that followed the operation, my father made what appeared to be a miraculous recovery, and by late December my parents made their annual winter retreat to their apartment in New Smyrna Beach, Florida. A month later, however, I received a telephone call in the middle of the night from my mother. My father had just had a devastating stroke and she wanted me to come to Florida immediately. Early that morning I arrived at Halifax Hospital in Daytona Beach and found my father lying paralyzed in the intensive care ward. Intravenous tubes, which hung from bottles above him, were injected into his arms.

After a discussion with the attending physician, it was agreed that Pop should have a head scan performed. It was possible that the stroke was caused by the malignancy infiltrating the brain. Soon, the results of the head scan came in: Five areas of my father's brain showed infiltration of cancer. That night my father was flown by air ambulance back to Philadelphia. He was taken to Jefferson Hospital where the following day he had his brain irradiated. Miraculously, he regained control over his arms and hands. More importantly, he was mentally lucid and seemed ready to stage another comeback. His courage buoyed my mother and me. We were still hoping for a miracle; meanwhile, I kept silent on what I believed his chances were. He was discharged from Jefferson Hospital, and my parents returned to their home in Long Beach Island, New Jersey. By spring the brain cancer had reemerged, and Pop began a slow and unmerciful decline. Since then I had been trying to make him comfortable and help my mother cope with the enormous strain of watching her husband die. These had not been easy times for my parents, nor for me.

The ringing of the silverware against the china plates brought me back to the restaurant and Bob Cathcart's question. "He's not doing well, Bob," I said. "I'm afraid it's just a matter of time before we'll have to bring him back to the hospital. Soon he'll need a lot more care than he's getting out on Long Beach Island."

"How's your mother taking all of this, Tony?" Bob asked.

"She's holding up well—as well as can be expected. My mother has always been the strongest member of the family."

Bob and I talked about other things—his family, Pennsylvania Hospital, politics. It wasn't until after the meal was finished and we were enjoying dessert that I mentioned—almost in passing—that I had fallen off my bicycle that morning and was suffering from an inflamed and painful testicle. I didn't mention the back pain. But as our conversation moved on to other topics, I reminded myself again of my appointment the next week with my internist.

On Wednesday morning, May 31, 1978, I arrived at my office and immediately went to the radiology department, where I had several x-rays taken of my chest and back; blood and liver tests were also performed. That previous summer I had contracted serum hepatitis after being pricked with a needle that had been used to treat a patient with the same disease. Since then, my liver functions had not returned to normal.

After the tests were done, I returned to my office to take on the day's work. Before I addressed the pile of papers waiting on my desk, I plugged in the heating pad and wedged it between my back and the chair. The pain was getting worse.

Later that morning, the chairman of our radiology department, Dr. Anthony Renzi, phoned me and said, "Tony, how do you feel?"

"I feel fine," I said. "What's up?"

"Well, there's something abnormal about your chest x-ray," said Renzi. "Why don't you come and have a look."

I got up from my desk and hurried up to radiology.

When I arrived, Tony Renzi put my chest x-rays on the lighted view box and I saw a large mass in the left side of my chest. At first it looked as if I had a large tumor in my left lung. Renzi and I discussed the x-rays, and as we did I became strangely aware of my left lung. My breathing had gotten noticeably shorter and my mouth was dry. I resisted the impulse to loosen my tie. In light of the x-rays, Renzi recommended that I have a bone scan performed immediately. I agreed.

Within an hour, I was back in radiology, where Renzi and his assistant injected a radioactive dye into my veins. I then had to wait three hours for the dye to spread throughout my body, after which a machine similar to a Geiger counter was suspended above me to determine how the dye reacted in my body. In the case of a person with cancer, the dye collects in large quantities wherever there is cancerous tissue. When the scanner is held over an area of the body where the dye has collected, the machine sends out a loud and rapid clicking sound. In the case of a person free of any tumors, however, the dye does not collect, but is spread homogenously throughout the body until it is largely eliminated through the urine. In this case, the machine clicks out a low, monotonous beat, since it doesn't detect any nests of cancer cells.

Three hours after I had had the radioactive dye injected into my veins, I lay down on the narrow table beneath the bone scan. I hoped to hear a low, monotonous click, indicating that the bone scan had found nothing abnormal.

I was naked, except for the inadequate hospital gown. I was cold and terribly nervous, and despite my efforts at self-control my body shivered as if I were lying on a block of ice. The massive machinery that would determine my fate loomed above me. The sensitive end of the bone scan is the size and shape of a snare drum. The drum faces down on the patient and is moved over each area of the body by the physician in charge. It is held in place by two heavy metal arms that are attached to a stand, all of which are connected to a computer that records the reactions of the bone scan. Built into the computer is an oscilloscope, or monitor, which provides an x-raylike picture of how the radioactive dye is reacting in the body. The doctor can actually see whether the dye is gathering in clumps in certain areas of the body, or whether it is spread evenly throughout the body.

I lay there looking up at the drum suspended above me. Two lines crossed one another at the center of the drum, like cross hairs on a rifle sight. As I lay there, I cast some feeble thoughts toward heaven, making deals with the Almighty. Renzi was ready, and just before he turned on the machine I reminded myself—in an effort to steady my nerves—that doctors don't get sick.

He threw the switch on the bone scanner, and like some massive creature that had just been woken up, it responded with a slow, desultory clicking sound, apparently picking up stray radioactive particles in the air. The scanner's sensory drum was placed over my head and suddenly the clicking sound shifted from a low, sporadic beat to a wild and terrifying machine-gun fire. My heart seemed to be keeping pace with it. My skin was suddenly galvanized by a wave of adrenalin and body heat. I took a quick look over at the monitor and saw to my disbelief what looked like a black spot at the top of my head. Renzi moved the machine down to my right shoulder, and after a brief pause in the clicking, the manic beat started again. It was the same over my sternum, my back, and the left side of my rib cage. I withdrew into a state of shock, but the sound of the clicks seemed to follow me inward. It was as if the clicking sound was taking place deep within the center of my brain. My whole mind and all of my senses were focused on those hideous clicks. They were cancer cells made audible.

After the bone scan was concluded, I got up from the table and wanted to vomit. Somehow my stomach held on while Renzi and I went over the test results. According to the bone scan, I had cancerous lesions in my skull, my left sixth rib, my right shoulder, sternum, and back. More x-rays were taken and somehow I dressed and made my way back to my office. Later, Tony Renzi came down to my office and tried to console me. I could see the deep concern in his round eyes and wide mouth. He appeared stiff, as if he wanted to exhale a long breath but couldn't.

"Tony, really, I don't think we can make any conclusions based on the bone scan," he said to me. "There's a chance it could have been reacting to some benign activity in bone tissue. We really won't know for sure until you have a biopsy. Please, let's not jump to any conclusions until we know for sure. Okay, Tony?"

"Okay," I mumbled. I could barely hear my own voice through the haze of my shock and the distant drone of clicks still going off in my mind.

The following morning, I took all of my test results to my physician. Dr. Sheldon Lisker is an internist as well as an oncologist, a doctor who specializes in the diagnosis and treatment of cancer. Sheldon has been my physician and friend since the late 1960s. He is a man of rare talents. While he maintains a large practice as both an internist and an oncologist, he also teaches medicine at the University of Pennsylvania Medical School and is chairman of Graduate Hospital's oncology and hematology departments. He is a dynamic and articulate man who has a wide view not only of medicine, but of literature and philosophy. He is in his early forties, about five feet eleven inches tall, and slightly overweight, which gives him a somewhat stocky appearance. His dark hair is combed straight back, revealing a receding hairline. The dominant characteristic about Sheldon's face — apart from his metal-framed glasses — is an expression that is at once compassionate yet curious about the person he is addressing. One can almost read concern and expectation in Sheldon Lisker's face, as if he were waiting for the patient himself to give the doctor the answer to the problem.

Sheldon examined me and paid particular attention to the swollen right testicle, which by now was abnormally hard. We then sat down and discussed the tests together. In addition to the bone scan, x-rays, and the hardened testicle, the blood tests revealed that my alkaline phosphatase levels were sharply elevated; my liver function tests were also abnormal, continuing in the same pattern that had been established the previous summer when I had contracted hepatitis. He then took my bone scan results, which provided x-raylike pictures, and put them on the lighted view box for examination.

That can't be me in those x-rays, I thought to myself.

"Tony," Sheldon said abruptly. "After looking at all of this, I have to tell you that I think you have either a testicular or prostatic carcinoma. There's a good chance that the cancer has spread to the other parts of your body — the skull, shoulder, sternum, rib, and spine — as indicated by the bone scan. I think you should have that testicle biopsied immediately. We should also have a biopsy done on the prostate gland."

Sheldon and I then sat down and discussed the possibilities further. There were a couple of incongruities in my case that did not fit into the classic pattern for either prostatic or testicular cancer. Testicular cancer usually does not spread to the bone, whereas my bone scan clearly indicated some type of bone lesions. On the other hand, prostatic cancer does not usually afflict Caucasian men in my age group. White males generally do not contract cancer of the prostate until they reach their late fifties. This was not a reassuring sign, however. Prostatic cancer in men under fifty is a much different, and far more perilous, disease. For reasons not yet fully understood, prostatic cancer spreads more rapidly in younger men and often kills its victim within two or three years after diagnosis. Men above the half-century mark with metastatic lesions to their bones can fare much better, sometimes living as long as five years; in rare instances, older men have been known to live even longer.

Sheldon tried to console me, but both of us knew that if the biopsy proved positive I probably wouldn't see my fiftieth birthday.

Sheldon Lisker's office is very near my home. When I left him, I walked to Rittenhouse Square. It was May 31, a warm and elegant spring day. The park benches were all occupied by people eating their lunches in the shadows of the tall trees. An occasional wind passed through the trees. Perfect sailing weather, I thought. An artist was displaying his works in one corner of the square. I browsed his collection and spotted an oil painting of two tennis players that I immediately wanted to buy. I was about to ask the artist for a price when, suddenly, the thought that I had been trying desperately to repress spilled over the walls of my consciousness. You're going to die, my mind cried out. What's the point? I quickly turned on my heel and hurried home.

That afternoon I went back to my office, hoping the work would occupy my mind. There was still the inspection approaching, I told myself. When I got there I called Dr. John Prehatny, our chairman of the department of surgery, to arrange to have the testicle and prostate gland biopsied. I would have to have the testicle removed. I would also have a transrectal biopsy of the prostate, a procedure that would remove some tissue from the prostate gland. That tissue, along with the testicle, would be examined for possible traces of cancer. John and I agreed to do the operation on Tuesday. I then made arrangements to check into Methodist as a patient on Monday afternoon. After I finished talking with John, I tried to plunge into my work; however, the effort was in vain. At five I went home to the emptiness of my apartment.

I knew that if I stayed alone in my apartment that night I would go out of my mind by morning. I needed to get away from Philadelphia, from the intensity and confusion of the city. I needed some solitude, a place to think, to prepare myself for what was coming. I also wanted to see my parents on Long Beach Island, New Jersey. I would be checking into the hospital on Monday and I wasn't sure how long it would be before I would see them again. I rented a car and began the two-hour drive. As I drove, I thought about the surgery I would undergo and tried to decide which fate was worse: that of knowing what was ahead or not knowing; I wished I didn't know.

By now the back pain was acute and rapidly getting worse. I felt as if a rusty spike were being driven into my spine. The pain radiated from a point in the center of my back and moved laterally across my rib cage to the sternum. It also moved up and down my spine, so that no matter how I stood or sat, I could not get any relief. It seemed to permeate every cell of my body, and at its peak it gripped my consciousness like a mailed fist.

I had begun taking aspirin and other painkillers by the mouthful. The analgesics provided only short-term relief, however, and I was left fighting the pain for long periods of time until I could safely take the next dose of painkillers. Most of my waking hours were spent contemplating my next pill.

As I drove to Long Beach Island, the spike dug itself deeper into my back. I told myself that I would begin taking a narcotic pain reliever when I returned to the hospital on Monday. As a certified anesthesiologist, I knew the full range of pain relievers available to me. Percodan would be best, I decided. At least for now.

Driving along Route 70 through New Jersey, I felt bitter over the ironic turn my life had taken. Just two days earlier, my mind had been consumed by the coming inspection and the success I was about to derive from it. I was certain that the trustees' doubts of me would vanish with the arrival of the inspection team's report. I would be fully installed at the helm of Methodist Hospital. The news had been so sudden. I felt cheated, somehow.

These feelings of failure and defeat were directly opposite to what I was used to feeling about my life. I had always felt blessed by life. I lived as if fate had made a promise to me. I had come to expect success.

Judging from the circumstances of my birth, one would have hardly guessed such a thing. I was born in an Italian ghetto in Perth Amboy, New Jersey, a city not far from the Jersey shore, known chiefly for the fact that it is the southernmost point of the great concrete and carbon-stained strip that runs north to Newark. It is this carnival of neon, asphalt, smokestacks, and broken glass that one sees when driving along the famed New Jersey Turnpike, a stretch of road that has almost single-handedly ruined the state's image.

When I was two, my parents bought a house in Highland Park, a small town in the central part of the state. Highland

Park is a sleepy, bedroom community, a half hour's train ride from New York City and walking distance from Rutgers University, in New Brunswick. It is in New York and at the college that many of the residents of Highland Park are employed. I grew up in a white, two-story wood-framed house, located in a quiet, residential neighborhood.

My parents were both of Italian descent, though they didn't speak the language much at home. They rarely argued in my presence, maintaining the old standard that when one was angry one kept silent—for days at a time, if necessary. On the whole, they were well matched and happy.

My father was the family's sole breadwinner. He worked for the New Brunswick News Agency, which distributed newspapers and magazines throughout New York and New Jersey. He rose to management level within the business and was well paid, especially by the standards of the Depression period. We were never in want that I could remember. He was a quiet man, who was a balancing and peacemaking force in the family. Although there were only the three of us—I was their only child—his diplomatic skills were often needed to settle the many heated arguments between my mother and me.

In my youth, he seemed forever buried in a newspaper or book, or leaving for work. He was handy around the house and was usually involved in some household project. Apart from his job, he had two loves outside the family: fishing and the church. On Saturdays he would often get up before the sun rose and drive to the Jersey shore to join a party boat. Later in the day, he would come home in a great whirlwind of excitement, full of fish stories and fish. On Sunday he was in church. He was very active in the church, not only going to Mass every Sunday and often during the week, but also involved in the many local church organizations and parish activities. My father was a Catholic, with an enormous faith that seemed to keep him on an even keel, no matter how emotional Mother and I would get. He was like a rudder in a storm; I can't remember him raising his voice in anger.

He liked to take day and weekend trips in the car. During the war years, we owned a 1939 Plymouth. We often drove to New York and a couple of times even made trips to Chicago and the West Coast. He loved to drive; it seemed to make him more conversational and outgoing.

I grew up feeling a certain remoteness about my father. I didn't like to fish, and my only link with the church was fear; for many years this was enough to keep me going to Mass every Sunday, but it didn't make me curious about what the church was all about, or what my father saw in it. It was not until I was older and more mature that I developed a curiosity about my father. And it was not until he was retired that I really got to know him.

My relationship with my mother was very different. I am convinced that had circumstances been different or had she been born a man, my mother would have been some kind of civic or business leader. She was the driving force behind the family, with more energy and determination than anyone I've ever met. Until I was ten, my mother was grossly overweight. At four feet eleven inches, she looked heavier than she actually was. Then one day, before my eleventh birthday, my mother—in typical fashion—announced a decision she had made: "I'm going on a diet, and I'm going to lose this weight," she said in a moderate, but self-assured tone. You could always tell when my mother meant what she said. She understated it.

In 1941, there were no reducing diets of the kind that we have today. So she devised her own plan: for a time, she simply stopped eating. And when she resumed she ate only small portions of food, usually vegetables. I used to needle her about how long she would stick to her diet. "You'll be eating everything in sight in a week," I kept telling her. But she didn't. Within a few months my mother was a different woman—a size five. From then on, she dressed smartly and always looked attractive. It was obvious that my father was proud of her.

Everything my mother gave her attention to was managed in the same orderly and determined way—the family finances, vacations, and most of all, the life and goals of her only son.

She wanted me to be successful and believed that education was my only chance. Any deviation I made from a straight A average sent off an alarm in her head. She was continually pushing me to study hard and read. However, it soon became apparent to both of us that I had inherited her strong will. When our wills diverged, as they often did, we clashed like a pair of rams.

Yet, by the time I reached high school I had become intellectually ambitious. While my friends measured their worth by the number of friends they had or by their competence in athletics, I measured mine by my grades and by the approval I received in school. I was always comparing myself to the students at the top of the class; I had to be as good or better than they were. And I usually was.

One day, while I was still in my freshman year of high school, my mother and I were in the kitchen. I was doing my homework and she was preparing dinner. Out of the blue, she announced another one of her decisions in her understated way. "You're going to become a doctor," she said.

At the time I had my heart set on becoming a teacher and following in the footsteps of my uncle, who taught high school Spanish and was regarded as the family intellectual.

For the next couple of years my mother and I fought over my future. In my junior year of high school, she went so far as to invite the guidance counselor to dinner to talk me into majoring in biology and premed in college in order to go to medical school after graduation. That night my mother and I argued vehemently, with the guidance counselor humiliated and trying to make peace between us. Later, Mom and I laughed uproariously about the incident.

Yet, when I got to college I did major in biology and premed. I attended Rutgers University and graduated magna cum laude. I was accepted at Hahnemann Medical College in Philadelphia and, four years later, graduated as a doctor. Hartford Hospital was the next stop; there I studied anesthesia and, shortly after completing the two-year course, entered the U.S. Air Force for a two-year stint. In 1962, I was discharged and went to work at Pennsylvania Hospital in Philadelphia. Two years later, I went to Methodist.

For the next twelve years, I enjoyed and drew great satisfaction from my job. But by the winter of 1976 my career had reached a plateau, which is to say it was going nowhere: I was burned out. I had been chairman of the department of anesthesiology, making more money than I needed, and there seemed to be no higher goal in my field to strive for. Strangely enough, I had begun to have some vague reluctance about injecting such massive dosages of drugs into patients in order to bring about anesthesia. I realized that this was necessary if operations were to be performed humanely, but this logic didn't seem to alleviate my growing sense of doubt. Probably this doubt sprang more from my desire to get out of anesthesia than from any sensitivity to the patient. At the same time, I plunged into a midlife crisis. My career was my life; when my work began to lose its luster and excitement, my entire existence seemed to become drab and fruitless. I needed a change, and I thought it might be to hospital administration.

In the summer of 1977, I got the opportunity to attend the Harvard Business School and School of Public Health's Health Systems Management Program. After I completed the program, I returned to Methodist hoping to assume an administrative position there or at some other hospital.

However, by that time the Board of Trustees had become disenchanted with the current administrator and I was approached about replacing him. I accepted the offer.

How ironic, I thought as I drove the car onto Highway 72 — the last leg of my trip to Long Beach Island — I was nearly at the summit. I thought I had Methodist and my whole career firmly in hand.

I arrived at my own house at Long Beach Island just before 8 P.M. As I got out of the car and walked toward the front door I could smell the salt air coming off the sea; it felt good to be there. When I got into the house, I went immediately into the kitchen and took some Darvon for my back. I then went upstairs and took a long hot shower, letting the water beat against my back to relieve the pain.

After I got out of the shower, I put on a robe and went downstairs to the living room and poured myself a tall V.O. I took the bottle and the glass back upstairs and placed them next to my chair outside on the sun deck. I then went back inside and put the Bach B Minor Mass on the stereo. I left the sliding door open so I could listen to the music while I sat on the chaise longue outside. I took a long swallow of whisky and I looked up at the stars.

The night was clear and infinite. From where I was sitting, I could see the moonlight glistening off the swells in the ocean. The gloom of death hung over me like a poisonous cloud. The suddenness of it all still had me reeling. It was as if I had awaked Thursday morning and walked into the wrong life. There was still a sense of living in a dream, as if reality had not caught up with me. I took another mouthful of whisky. I was counting on the liquor to put me to sleep.

I considered my chances of surviving. They were painfully slim. Both testicular and prostatic cancer with metastatic lesions to the bone are extremely lethal diseases. Testicular cancer is the more virulent of the two, often claiming the victim's life within six months to a year. Prostatic cancer with bone lesions is most often fatal as well, particularly in men my age. My only hope was that the bone scan was reacting to benign activity in bone tissue. Yet, even if this were the case, there were still the blood tests, which indicated the presence of cancer as well. I had to hope for the long shot — that my cancer was localized in the prostate, which could be treated successfully by removing the prostate gland.

I was afraid the cancer might spread to the brain and cause a stroke. I thought of my father and so many other stroke victims I had known. I took another long swallow of whisky. God, not that.

How did my father cope? His faith in God gave him incredible courage, the extent of which I had only now begun to realize. Although I had grown up going to church on Sundays, I was only a nominal Catholic. I attended Mass throughout my four years in medical school, but as soon as I graduated, I left the church. Through the sixties I was indifferent to matters of the spirit. I got caught up in my career. In the early seventies, my interest in religion was rekindled and I began to attend the Unitarian church; I stayed through most of the seventies. I went to services every week and eventually was asked to become a member of the church's Board of Trustees. I served on the board a few years and liked going to church. I realized during those years that there was a deep spiritual need within me that had to be addressed. It was not until much of the fear I had experienced in my youth had passed away that I was able to recognize my own desire for spiritual nourishment. During my years at the Unitarian church, I had a hunger for intellectual arguments for the reality of God. I had no faith, but a desire to be convinced. I was fascinated by such writers as Reinhold Niebuhr, Dietrich Bonhoeffer, and Paul Tillich. I also engaged in great intellectual debates with the minister at the First Unitarian Church, Reverend Victor Carpenter.

But, in 1977, the back pain had become so great that I could no longer sit for an hour in those stiff wooden pews without great discomfort. I stopped going to church altogether. I still had no faith when I left. Intellectual arguments all seem to descend to a competition of words, and there always seems to be someone of the opposing point of view who is a little more eloquent than the one before him. My father did not argue his faith; he practiced it quietly.

I emerged from my reverie to notice that the Bach had long since stopped. I got up and turned the record over, refilled my glass, and returned to my chair. I listened to the Agnus Dei. One thing my father and I had in common was that we both liked good music.

The pain in my back was starting to return. I could feel that spike starting to awaken and grow angry. I thought of taking some sleeping pills but decided that I had had too much whisky for that. I was not ready for suicide yet. I hoped the whisky would bring sleep on soon.

I spent the next hour thinking of what I would do the following day. I knew I would have to see my parents, who were living five miles south of my house. I had decided not to tell them that I, too, had cancer. My mother could not cope with my dying alongside my father. I would tell my mother that I'd be away at meetings in Chicago for a few weeks, and that she shouldn't call the hospital for me. I would tell her that I'd call when I got back. I'd have my staff go along with this charade. They'd understand.

My hope was that I would hang on at least until after my mother had recovered from my father's death. Then I would tell her of my own condition.

There was also the hospital to take care of. I had already called the chairman of the board, Robert Bent, and asked to see him the following day. Bob had a house at Long Beach

Island not far from my own. I planned to tell him of my disease, the state of the hospital, and how we would fare with the coming inspection.

I got up from my chair, turned off the stereo, and, sufficiently numb from the alcohol, managed to go upstairs to bed, where I fell into a fitful sleep.

I got up early Saturday morning and walked a couple of miles along the beach. It was a cloudless morning, the sun fresh and young. The sand was off-white and it was still early enough in the season so that the beach was relatively free of litter. Long Beach Island has a beautiful stretch of beach, with many large, old wooden houses that look out over the ocean. As I walked in the shallow surf, sea gulls buzzed over me and then flew out to sea.

Later, I came back to the house and called Bob Bent to set a time to get together. At noon, I went to his house, which was lovely and sat right on the beach looking out on Barnegat Bay. When I entered the house and saw Bob's wife, Edith, I was immediately horrified by her condition. She had just had a stroke and was now paralyzed; she could hardly talk. Edith had been a very bright woman, who loved to read. To my disbelief, the stroke had left her almost blind, so that reading was out of the question. She looked incredibly frail, as if her bones could not support the weight of her dress. Her skin and hair were both gray, and her eyes teared; she looked as if she had been standing too long in the wind.

Bob, a big man who must have played football in his youth, seemed to sense my discomfort. He suggested that we go out on the sun deck where we could talk. When we got outside, I told Bob in very detached terms the details of my condition. As I spoke, I was surprised at how impersonal I could be about myself. (This later turned out to be the very persona I adopted whenever I spoke to friends or relatives about my cancer.) Bob listened intently. When I finished, I told him what my perceptions were of the hospital staff, and what else needed to be done before we underwent the inspection; I also told him whom I planned to appoint as my replacement while I was recovering from surgery. We talked for about an hour and then he escorted me to my car. There he put his arm around me and wished me luck. I thanked him and left.

I dreaded where I had to go next. I tried to pull myself together and rehearse what I was about to tell my parents. I went over the plan several times before I arrived at their home. When I walked in, I saw my father sitting in one corner of the living room holding his head. The cancer in his skull had left him with intense headaches, something akin to migraines. On top of that, he was suffering from bone pain to such an extent that he had trouble lying down. The man was being crippled up like an old vine. I went over to him and put my arm around his shoulder. My mother then came into the room and the three of us talked. I tried to lighten my father's mood by making small jokes. He smiled and pretended to laugh. He didn't want to be pitied. My mother was dealing with the crisis by talking excessively. It was her way of burning up nervous tension.

We talked awhile longer and then I got my mother alone in the kitchen. I asked about Pop. He was managing, she said. Then I told her in very firm terms that I was going away for a few weeks. I would be in Chicago at meetings and I would call her the minute I returned. I would be very busy when I was gone so I couldn't call from Chicago. Don't call the hospital unless you have an emergency and want to relay a message to me, I told her. I'll be back soon; I'll come to Long Beach Island as soon as I get back.

We then joined my father, but I couldn't bear to stay and soon left.

I drove back to my house and then telephoned St. Francis Church, where my parents attended Mass. Father Thaddeus answered the telephone. He knew my parents and also knew my father was suffering from cancer.

"The reason I'm calling, Father, is because I'm dying of cancer also, and I'm going into the hospital to be operated on. My parents don't know this and I don't want them to. But while I'm in the hospital, I'd like you to look after them. They are very dear to me, and they need help. I can't give it to them. I need someone down here who can call me in case my father takes a bad turn. Will you do that for me?"

"Dr. Sattilaro," he said. "I'm utterly shocked by this tragedy. Of course I'll look after your parents and stay in touch with you. Is there anything I can do for you?"

"No, thank you. But I do appreciate your concern."

"Why don't you let me come by your house tomorrow. Would you let me do that? I'd like to talk with you," Father Thaddeus said.

"That will be fine," I told him. Suddenly, I looked forward to having someone to confide in.

"Thanks," I said and rang off.

It was another whisky and Darvon day. Luckily I got tired before I got too depressed and fell asleep. At about midnight, my mother called me. She was hysterical. "Your father is choking to death," she said. "Get down here, right away!"

I raced to my parents' house, burst into their room, and found my father gagging murderously. A few minutes later he coughed up a fist of mucus, which apparently had been lodged in his throat. I checked him and then his physician came by and examined him also. I tried to steady my parents, especially my mother, who I feared was approaching some kind of psychological breaking point. She talked excessively and she seemed to be creating new things to worry about by the minute. Her nervous tension made her hyperattentive to my father; she couldn't relax around him.

She was constantly asking him if he needed something; if he didn't want something to eat; if she couldn't do something to make him more comfortable.

"Mom, try to relax," I told her.

"I'll be all right. Don't worry. Everything's fine," she said.

After things calmed down, I left. I got into my car and rested my head on the steering wheel for a moment. How am I going to cope with all of this? I wondered. It can't go on much longer; one of us is going to collapse.

When I got home, I took some more pills and went to sleep.

The next day Father Thaddeus came by. We sat together on the deck of my house watching the sun glisten off the ocean, while the sea gulls dove for fish. We talked for a few hours about my cancer and my father's. We also talked about God, religion, and why I left the church. Father Thaddeus was a kind man, and a good listener.

That night I returned to Philadelphia. Bob Cathcart called and later dropped in to talk for a while. After he left, the phone rang; it was Father Thaddeus calling. He wanted to tell me that I'd be in his prayers along with my parents. I was touched by his gesture and thanked him.

The next morning I arrived at my office and conducted the regular staff meeting. After the meeting was concluded, I issued a memo to the staff stating that Joe Manson, the executive vice president, would act as chief executive officer in my stead. I didn't want any political warfare going on while I was being treated. I then called Joe into my office, where I went over with him what I expected to be done while I was out.

"There won't be any second-guessing from upstairs, Joe," I said. "I only ask that you keep me informed."

Joe tried to reassure me that I would be back to work in no time. After he left I attended to some last-minute work and then signed myself in as a patient. I then went upstairs to my room, got into my bedclothes, and into bed. I looked around the room, feeling increasingly desperate. It's come to this, I said to myself. I thought then that this was the beginning of the end.

Chapter 2

*T*HAT AFTERNOON, I sat up in my bed thinking of what would happen to me. They were grim thoughts. John Prehatny visited me to describe the operation; his words seemed to support my worst expectations. It would be a radical right inguinal dissection, which would remove my right testicle and all of the lymph nodes on the right side of my groin area. The nodes would be removed in order to protect against any further spread of the malignancy, assuming I had a testicular cancer. It would not be a long operation, perhaps two hours. It was not a particularly dangerous procedure, either, though that did little to comfort me. Despite the fact that I would not be left sterile, nor sexually impotent, I nevertheless had the feeling that my manhood was being ripped away.

After John left, I tried to come to grips with my fear and began to think of the many people I had seen come into that operating room. They all had the same expression on their faces: complete surrender. Most of them looked as if they were on the edge of death, if not from their illnesses, then from their fear.

Tomorrow I would see that operating team as a patient

sees them—masked and clad in their green gowns, looking professionally detached from humanity, the same way I had looked to so many other fearful people.

Lying there in my bed, I began to wonder when it was that I had stopped seeing patients as people. When did people become sick gall bladders, or ruptured appendixes, or cancerous lungs? My attitude, I realized, was partly a defense mechanism against experiencing on some vicarious level the patient's trauma. I had spent the last thirteen years of my life looking into the face of human terror. Like most people who work in hospitals, I had become calloused to the human condition, as much by the daily routine of seeing illness as by the need to keep from feeling the accumulated effects of the patient's agony. And so, when the patient was wheeled into the operating room, I withdrew into my professional shell. I didn't want to get involved with him or her on any level. Besides, in most cases, I had decided, the operations were minor and their fears unfounded.

The knowledge that my operation was minor did little to allay my fears.

Fortunately, I could not be alone to think for very long; it seemed that everyone in the hospital wanted to come by and wish me luck before I went for surgery the following day. There was a steady stream of visitors, and from what they told me, I would be well represented by their prayers in heaven that day and the next. After visiting hours had concluded, a nurse came into my room and gave me some medication to help me fall asleep.

The operation was to take place at 8 A.M. the next day. I awoke that Tuesday morning at six, got out of bed, showered, shaved, and waited. Gloom hung over me. I was convinced that they would find me riddled with cancer. My life was now completely out of my own hands. I wanted to slow time down, but just the opposite seemed to be happening. I was hurtling toward the unknown.

Soon, a very cheerful nurse hurried into my room and said, "We're ready to take you upstairs, Dr. Sattilaro." She then gave me some preoperative medication — atropine — which dried the saliva and mucus from my mouth and throat and kept them dry during the surgery. I got on the litter and was wheeled to the elevator, which took me up to the sixth floor and the pre-anesthesia waiting room. It is a long and narrow room, where six to eight litters are aligned head first against one wall, something like parked cars all parallel with their headlights pointing toward the curb. I was wheeled in and parked among several other patients, who were also waiting for operating rooms. A nurse came by, checked my name and numbers on my name bracelet, and then wrapped my head in a towel. She then checked to see if I was securely strapped onto the litter. Suddenly, John Prehatny came in from the operating room and bade me good morning. I was then wheeled into operating room number two.

The operating room is a mammoth chamber in battleship gray. The walls are covered with ceramic tile; the floors are made of a conductive material to channel static electricity out of the room. The ceiling is lined with fluorescent lights that shine down on the patient and the operating team. The room is almost futuristic, in that it is filled with ultramodern equipment and instruments. Yet, for all its high technology and surgical success stories, it is a joyless chamber that carries with it the heaviness and gloom of many deaths.

I was placed on a rubber mattress atop a metal bed, three feet wide and about six feet long. While Dr. Prehatny stood over me, the anesthetists prepared to give me anesthesia.

"Take good care of me," I told them.

The anesthetists then inserted a needle into my arm and the sodium pentothal flowed through the tube and into my veins. Ten seconds later, I was unconscious. The right testicle was removed and an inguinal dissection performed along with a transrectal biopsy of the prostate. The biopsy was done by taking a long hypodermic needle and inserting it through the rectum and into the prostate gland and withdrawing some tissue. That tissue, along with the right testicle, was then sent to the pathology laboratory, where it was examined for traces of cancer.

At about 11 A.M., I started to regain consciousness. As I woke, Reverend John Mcellhenny, the vice chairman of our Board of Trustees, and his wife, Nancy, were standing over me. My eyes opened and John bent down and kissed my forehead. I managed a faint smile and whispered something inaudible. John told me that he was on his way to the Annual Conference of the Methodist Church. He said that he had already requested the conference leadership to have the ministers at the gathering pray for me. I thanked him and fell back to sleep. Later, after I woke, the memory of his kiss and his request of the ministers touched me deeply, and for a moment I didn't feel so alone.

Such feelings of comfort were short-lived, however. The pain in my back seemed worse than ever; I also had a burning pain in my groin area as a result of the operation. On top of this, I had a raging fever that hovered around 104 degrees, a fringe benefit from the prostatic biopsy. When the biopsy was performed, the needle that was inserted through the rectum caused some feces to spill into the blood. This resulted in an infection and a fulminating fever. For the next four days I passed in and out of delirium, and when I wasn't delirious, I was filled with anger.

When my fever subsided and I was no longer in any danger from the infection, the biopsy results from the testicle and prostate came back. The testicle was clean; however, the prostate gland was filled with cancer.

On June 11, John Prehatny came into my room and told me that he would have to remove the left sixth rib to see if the cancer had spread to the other places indicated by the bone scan. I was hoping that the bone scan might have indicated some benign changes in the bone tissue, and not cancer. If this were the case, then my cancer would be localized in the prostate gland, which could be treated with surgery; I would have a good chance of living a long life. It was an unlikely possibility, but one that had to be explored. The only way to test the diagnosis of the bone scan was to examine one of the areas where the scan had indicated a tumor. The left sixth rib was the only place such an examination could be made.

"Okay, John," I said. "Let's do it tomorrow."

"I can't operate on you tomorrow, Tony," John said. "Tomorrow is your forty-seventh birthday. We'll do it the day after tomorrow."

On the following day, my staff paraded into my room with a large birthday cake and sang happy birthday to me. They all seemed merry and tried to lift me out of my gloom. I forced a smile, but inside I was desolate. My life hung by the remote chance that the bone scan was wrong. If it was right, and there was cancer in the rib, I knew I was finished, and all the birthday wishes in the world wouldn't change that.

When the party ended, I tried to rest. I was extremely nervous about the operation, for unlike the inguinal dissection, the removal of a rib, called a thoracotomy, was a serious and delicate surgical procedure. I was very worried that all would not go right. My many years in the operating room seemed to work against me; I was plagued by the memories of operations that went wrong. On top of this heightened concern was the feeling that I was living in a dreamlike state, in which my life was totally out of control. Clearly, much of this was due to the enormous amount of drugs I was taking, including morphine every four hours for the back pain, a variety of drugs for the surgery, and medication to help me sleep. All of this created a deep paranoia in me; I believed that some mistake would be made when I got to the operating room. I was particularly worried that the wrong rib would be taken out. In a panic, I called Tony Renzi and expressed my fears.

"If you feel that strongly about it, Tony," said Renzi, "then a half hour before you go upstairs to surgery I'll insert a hypodermic needle into the rib itself. That will assure you of getting the right rib operated on." I agreed with this and hung up. I spent the next hour thinking of other things that might go wrong.

I slept badly that night and woke up the next morning feeling as if I hadn't slept in days. After I was up a little while, a nurse came in and wheeled me on a litter to radiology. As I entered the x-ray room, I became cold and shook intensely.

There Tony Renzi put xylocaine, a local anesthetic, over the area of the left sixth rib and then plunged a hypodermic needle into the bone. He placed a dressing around the needle and I was taken to the pre-anesthesia waiting room. A nurse came out of the operating room, checked my name bracelet, and then wrapped my head in a towel. There were six other patients in the room. I felt the urge to tell them that I was the guy who used to be in charge here. But, of course, that didn't matter; I was just another racked body.

John Prehatny came into the waiting room and said, "Okay, Tony, let's go." With that I was wheeled into the operating room and placed once again on the table. The sodium pentothal rushed into my veins. Just before I went off to sleep, I asked the operating team again to take good care of me. Then I fell into a bottomless sleep.

I had participated in this operation many times before. Once asleep from the anesthetic, the patient is given an injection of curare, a South American Indian poison, which is used to paralyze the entire body. The patient immediately stops breathing. The anesthesiologist then takes an endotracheal tube and inserts it into the windpipe through the larynx. He then attaches a long rubber tube to the endotracheal tube, which he hooks up to a machine that breathes for the patient, usually fifteen to twenty times per minute. At the same time, anesthetic is being injected into the patient's body through the intravenous, as well as through the endotracheal tube in the form of gas.

The patient is placed on his side and scrubbed, after which the body is draped so that only the portion of the body to be operated on is exposed. Electrocardiogram electrodes are placed on the arms and legs.

When all this is finished, the surgeon comes into the room, after scrubbing up outside. A nurse then helps him dry his hands and get into a sterile surgical gown. She then holds up a pair of sterile gloves, into which the surgeon plunges his hands. The whole front of the surgeon's body is then sterile. He is now ready to operate.

At the foot of the bed is the instrument table, and surrounding the table is the operating team, which is usually made up of seven or eight people in the case of a thoracotomy. The team consists of the surgeon, his first assistant—usually a senior resident in training—a second assistant, who is often a medical student, a scrub nurse, who assists the surgeon and handles the instruments, a circulating nurse, who will assist the team in getting whatever additional equipment or instruments are necessary, and the anesthetist and his assistant. In some cases, a second first assistant is present, also. When everyone is ready, the surgeon begins the operation by saying "Scalpel."

The surgeon takes the scalpel and, using only the weight of the knife, runs the blade across the body over the area of the rib. The long, elliptical incision at first seems to have made only a hairline scratch in the skin. However, in a moment blood and fat globules appear and the deep incision widens. At that point, an electrical cauterizer, known as a bovie, is run across the edge of the incision, burning the small blood vessels shut. The smell of burning flesh hangs in the air for a few minutes until the ventilation clears it away. The larger vessels, which have not been burned closed, are then clamped. After the initial incision has been made, the surgeon makes another, deeper cut through the muscle and to the bone. His associate then ties off the larger blood vessels. Once the ribs are exposed, metal retractors are inserted between the ribs and then cranked open until the rib cage is spread apart. On the in-breath, the large, pink, beautiful lung expands into the open area between the ribs, and then collapses with the out-breath. Throughout the operation the lung continues to expand and contract in and out of the rib opening with each pump of gas from the anesthesia machine.

With the rib cage exposed, the surgeon examines the area for a tumor. When Dr. Prehatny looked at my left sixth rib, he saw a large tumor, the size of a plum, growing out of the rib. He then searched the area to see if the tumor had spread to any other ribs, or to the lung. Apparently, it had not.

To remove the rib, the surgeon uses a pair of rib cutters, with long handles and short cutting nose, similar to the tool used to cut hedges. Sometimes the rib will not yield to the cutters, and a saw is used.

After the rib has been severed at both ends, the retractors are removed and the surgeon begins to stitch the incision closed. The rib is sent to the pathology lab, where it is checked for malignancy. At this point in the surgery, the breathing tube is detached from the gas machine and attached to an air bag that is controlled by the anesthetist's hand. When the surgeon is ready, the anesthetist gives the bag a hard squeeze, thus expanding the lung to its maximum capacity, and driving out most of the air that has seeped in between the lung and the chest wall during the operation. The anesthetist continues breathing for the patient until the operation is concluded.

The surgeon sews the incision closed, except for a small

area of the chest, about an inch wide, in which a tube is inserted into the chest wall. This tube allows any remaining air that has been trapped between the chest and the lung during the operation to escape. While one end of the tube is inside the chest wall, the other end is placed in a bottle containing water. When the patient breathes, any air that has remained inside the chest wall is pushed out and down the tube into the bottle of water, where it bubbles and escapes. The water also prevents any air from coming back up from the other end of the tube. The tube is long enough so that gravity keeps the water from being sucked back into the chest wall. This tube is kept in the chest for about a week after the operation.

At the end of the surgical procedure, a new round of drugs are injected into the patient, relieving him or her of the paralyzing effects of the curare.

After John Prehatny finished stitching me up, I was wheeled into the recovery room, where I spent the next hour. The operation had taken about three hours. Later, I was taken back to my room, where the anesthetic finally wore off. It was early afternoon when I began to awaken.

The spring sun was pouring in on me from the bay window of my room. I could see the blue sky and some thick pillows of cumulus clouds; an occasional bird flew by. My consciousness was coming back in stages, and I began to feel increasingly like a prisoner. Suddenly, I realized that my movements were restricted by a loose, cloth belt around my chest to protect me from inadvertently pulling the chest tube out of my side. I settled back and continued looking out the window. It seemed like an eternity before I felt the massive pain coming from my chest and back. A nurse came into my room and gave me some medication and I fell back to sleep.

When I awoke again, I was anxious about the results of the biopsy and asked the nurse several times to have the pathologist call me. It would be days before the biopsy was completed, I was told. All I could do was wait.

I spent the next couple of days passing in and out of sleep, as visitors came with flowers. The staff at Methodist was very generous, but eventually people had trouble moving around the room for the flowers, so I had an attendant pass them out to other patients on the floor.

All I could think about was the pathologist's report. Each day I phoned to the laboratory to find out what stage the biopsy was in, and each day I got the same response: No answer yet.

Meanwhile, the State Health Department's inspection team came through the hospital. Methodist passed the inspection easily and there was a very complimentary report from the inspectors to the Board of Trustees. I read the report with little enthusiasm. For me, it was all perversely irrelevant. I was pleased in some detached way that we had passed. I was very loyal to Methodist and was committed to seeing the institution continue in high standing. Yet, so much had changed in so short a time. Two weeks before, I was fighting for my ego. That day, I was battling for my life. Lying in that bed, racked with pain, and holding on to the small hope that I would survive this incredible nightmare, I started to look back at my life from a new perspective. I had never before appeared so small to myself. I tossed the report to the foot of the bed and looked out the window at the passing clouds.

The weekend came and went and still no word from pathology. Finally, on Monday morning, John Prehatny came into my room and sat on the end of my bed. Before he spoke, he just looked at me, perhaps to give me a chance to read the bad news on his face and brace myself.

"I've got a lot of problems telling you this, Tony," John said. "But the rib is loaded with cancer."

John was silent for a moment while I absorbed the impact of his words. They blew the strength right out of me. His meaning was clear: The bone scan had reacted to cancerous lesions, which meant that the tumors in my rib, sternum, shoulder, spine, and skull were all malignant. Any hope that I was holding on to suddenly vanished.

"I'm disappointed, John," I said. I couldn't stop the tears from coming.

"I've talked to Sheldon Lisker, Tony, and he agrees that we should take off the other testicle."

Removal of both testicles, called an orchiectomy, was a standard treatment for cancer of the prostate. By removing the testicle, one eliminates the male hormone, testosterone. If left in, testosterone speeds the growth of the malignancy; removal of testosterone tends to slow the spread of the cancer cells, and thus extends the patient's life. Usually, an orchiectomy is used in combination with daily doses of estrogen, the female hormone, in an effort to further stem the growth of the tumor and alleviate pain.

John proceeded to tell me that if we went ahead with this third operation, I would very likely not be capable of having sex, or even procreation. On the other hand, if we didn't do the operation, my condition would rapidly degenerate and the pain would get even worse.

"Okay," I said. "Let's do it tomorrow. I want to be out of bed by noon tomorrow and out of the hospital by Saturday."

"If you're fit, that's fine with me," John said.

The following morning I went up to the operating room for the third time in three weeks. The second testicle was removed. This time it was a much simpler operation. The surgeon opened the scrotum and cut off the remaining testicle. The lymph nodes were not touched. The surgery required about an hour. I was back in my room by eleven.

The anesthetic wore off around noon. For a while, I just sat there in bed thinking. I was no longer whole. I felt less than human. What was I anymore? I knew what I was. For a while longer I just sat there and sobbed. Then I got out of the bed and headed for the bathroom. Fear was in me like an electric current. I didn't want to know but I had to. I removed some of the bandages. My hands shook. I was able to urinate normally and felt some small gratitude for it. I had had some irrational fear that I might have lost everything. Then the fear got stronger. I reached down, touched my leg, and then the emptiness. A rush of shock and anger filled my stomach and swelled into my chest. Suddenly I was consumed by a cloud of emotion. I bent down and knelt on the floor.

"No, dear God, no..." I cried.

Several hours later, after I had become relatively composed, I sat in my bed thinking of the many things I would have to take care of in the months ahead. For the first time in a week, I thought of my parents. How would I handle them? I wondered. There was the hospital to take care of also. How much longer would I be able to work?

I would talk to Sheldon Lisker about my condition when I got out of the hospital, but I knew well in advance how grave my circumstances were. I was losing my life in great chunks. The fear of a stroke was always nearby and threatening. In my darker moments, I pictured myself in a wheelchair, staring off into space, with that same blank stare that Edith Bent had. That stare seemed impossible to shake from my mind. It reminded me of a burned-out tenement, with only its shell remaining.

Later that day, Brian Kopke, my minister at the First Unitarian Church of Philadelphia, came by my room to console me. Brian is young—in his middle thirties—blond, bearded, and built like a bear. He always reminded me of an overweight John the Baptist.

Brian sat down on the chair next to my bed and tried to get me to focus upward at heaven. "Ask for God's help, Tony," he said. "You don't have to bear this by yourself."

"I'm going to die, Brian," I told him. "But not before I've gone through a lot of pain, the way my father's dying."

"No one knows when they're going to die, Tony. That's up to God. Ask for God's help now. Don't shut God out."

Despite Brian's loving pleas, I never felt more alone and helpless in my life. All I could think about was death coming on me. I was like a man drowning; Brian wanted me to look for God in the water, but all I could think about was a life preserver. Despite my inability to respond to him spiritually, Brian visited me every day while I was in the hospital and supported me through the difficult months ahead.

On Saturday, June 17, 1978, I returned home for what was scheduled to be six weeks of recuperation. On the following Monday, I visited Sheldon Lisker. We went over all the tests again, as well as the biopsies of the testicle, prostate, and rib. The diagnosis was that I had prostatic cancer, state IV (D), which meant that it had spread to several other parts of my body. Sheldon reviewed the data on prostatic cancer with me. None of the studies was encouraging.

The data varied, but at most only 15 to 25 percent of men with this disease survived five years with the standard treatment — orchiectomy and estrogens. There was nothing in the medical literature to suggest that a man of my age with a well-differentiated carcinoma of the prostate had any reason to hope to live longer. In fact, the literature indicated just the opposite: the odds were great that I would be dead well before the five years had passed.

We had no other course but to hope for the long shot. Perhaps the orchiectomy would slow the progress of the disease, or even send it into remission. We would know how effective the surgery was within six weeks. If the pain subsided, then the orchiectomy was working; if the pain didn't subside, then I would begin taking estrogens, the female hormone. Although the odds that this treatment would save me were small at best, the alternatives appeared utterly hopeless. If the estrogens and orchiectomy didn't work, my only hope seemed to rest on the remote chance that science would come up with a cure for cancer before 1981 or 1982. I was reminded that this was, after all, 1978, and medicine was struggling for a breakthrough. Something might happen, I told myself.

"How many years do I have left, Sheldon?"

"Tony," Sheldon said, "I think you have some years left. Don't ask me to be more specific than that, because I simply can't be. No physician can tell his patients how long they have to live. We can talk about populations, the average survival rates, epidemiological studies, but when it comes down to telling an individual how long he or she has to live—that's impossible."

Some years left, I said to myself. Judging by what we had already discussed, I took this to mean three years at the most. Over the next few months, I would come to realize that three years would be the outside figure any physician would give me. Some thought I could be dead within eighteen months.

"How long will I be able to work, Sheldon?" I explained the tenuous position I was in at Methodist and asked him if he felt I should resign now for the good of the hospital.

"No. You should work for as long as you possibly can," Sheldon said. "The worst thing you can do is stop working."

Sheldon and I had had many philosophical discussions in the past about how a doctor could best help a patient with a terminal illness. Sheldon was always of the belief that the physician should inform the patient of the gravity of the illness, but never make the judgment that the disease would be terminal in this particular patient's case. There was always the chance that for some medically unexplainable reason the patient might be able to pull through. One of the ways a patient could best help himself was to continue to feel of value, not only to himself, but to others. One of the best and easiest ways of doing this was to work.

I had never guessed that Sheldon would one day be having this discussion with me.

We talked about my back pain and agreed that I would begin taking Percodan, a narcotic pain reliever, for my back. After our discussion, I left his office and went home to contemplate my circumstances.

It would be four weeks before I returned to work. They were four tormented weeks. Pain became my protagonist. Everything I did was governed by it. It was worse than ever now and the thought occurred to me many times to simply jump off my terrace and end my life on the asphalt below. I found out quickly, however, that no matter how tormented I was, suicide was not an option for me.

Some of the credit for keeping me alive must surely go to the Percodan. I took a couple of Percodan tablets every six hours and the combination of pain relief and narcotic stimulation drove me to euphoric heights. After taking the pills, my problems seemed to fit into small boxes in my mind. I could then close the lids on those boxes and deal with each problem individually. Suddenly, my life was manageable; my problems were not insurmountable. I made plans for my future, at least what was left of it. There were still "some" years left — time to work, to accomplish a few important goals, to run a hospital. A rush of emotion would fill my heart. I'm alive now, I would say. Let tomorrow take care of itself. Besides, there will be more Percodan tomorrow, too. Life seemed cushioned. Somehow, things would work out, I thought.

Of course, the euphoria didn't last. After a couple of hours, the Percodan would wear off, and I would swing back toward the other end of the emotional spectrum. I came down hard. I became deeply depressed. The pain seemed worse every time I dropped from my euphoric heights and with it I became all the more disappointed and despondent.

On top of this, I also became deeply bitter. I had gone

into the hospital for the relief of the pain; when I emerged from the surgery, however, I still had the pain and it was worse than ever. The loss of my sexuality was a greater blow than any I had ever received in life. I was never so aware of the power of the sex drive until it was missing. There was suddenly a void inside of me that I could never fill. And every time I went to urinate or defecate, the empty scrotum hung there as a reminder that I had lost more than a part of my anatomy, even more than sex. I was the only son of John Sattilaro; it was an ignoble end to a proud lineage.

What made it all seem worse, however, was that I was alone so much of the time. I had an occasional telephone call or visitor—Bob Cathcart, Brian Kopke, friends from the hospital—but I was very much alone. During my twenty years in Philadelphia, I had come to love many people, but, sadly, I kept them at a distance; I never allowed anyone to come too close. Part of this was due to my overly ambitious nature. I had become too cautious, untrustful, and even suspicious of others. On top of this, I felt a deep need always to be in control, a compulsion that also kept me from allowing people to get too close to me. I wanted to be in a position where it was easy to say no. During those four weeks at home, I kept hearing the words of Thomas Merton ringing in my ears: "Only-sons make for solitary men."

These periods of despondency would last as long as two or three hours, since the Percodan often wore off well before I could safely take another round of pills. Had the Percodan not had several powerful side effects, I would probably not have observed the six-hour time limit between dosages. However, the drug made me extremely nauseated and caused me to vomit. The nausea was worse when I took the medication more frequently than was recommended. Thus, I was forced to decide which fate was worse: to suffer the excruciating pain in my back or to spend part of the day in the bathroom vomiting. I spent much of my time racked with pain, emotionally drained, and physically fatigued.

Yet, in a perverse way, the pain also had a beneficial side effect: It prevented me from dwelling on any one problem for too long.

And so, each day I was caught up in this manic-depressive cycle. I could chart the points in between, as I watched myself go from an intoxicated optimist to a hopeless depressive.

Besides the pain, one other subject did occupy center stage in my mind, however. That subject was death. When the Percodan began to wane and my euphoria had passed, the first thought to come to my mind was my own death.

How will it come? I wondered.

After I got home from the hospital, I sought refuge from my problems in various forms of escapism. I tried to read but, ironically, all I could concentrate on was that which preoccupied my mind: death. I read Elisabeth Kübler-Ross's *On Death and Dying,* Kathryn Kuhlman's *I Believe in Miracles,* and Carl Simonton's *Getting Well Again.* I also read some religious literature, hoping to make some sense out of my inscrutable fate, or at least find something that might help me transcend the agony of dying. I found some small solace in what I read, but nothing transcendent.

I watched a lot of television—from the morning game shows to the late night reruns. And I forced myself to get out of the house and walk. I knew, however, that if I was going to keep my sanity I would have to go back to work. After four weeks at home, I returned to the hospital on a part-time basis.

Chapter 3

THAT JULY, we began to plan a building program to rebuild and renovate the hospital laboratories, operating rooms, intensive care unit, and several other areas of the complex. It was a $20 million building project and there would be months of planning and fund raising ahead before we went before the appropriate local and state agencies for approval to build the facility. I viewed the project as just the challenge I needed to occupy my mind and plunged into the work of organizing our proposal.

Six weeks after the operations, there was still no reduction of the pain as a result of the orchiectomy. Dr. Lisker recommended that I begin a therapeutic estrogen challenge. At first I was given the estrogens intravenously and later took two milligrams orally each day. We hoped the estrogens, combined with the orchiectomy, would send the cancer into remission and reduce the pain, but throughout the months of July and August the pain persisted at a constant level. The narcotics provided me with the only relief I could get. In addition, there were no signs that the cancer was being halted.

By the end of July, I had sufficiently recovered from the

surgery to see my parents. I took a couple of days off from work and went to my house on Long Beach Island to try to get a suntan. I looked gaunt and pale; I had lost about ten pounds since the operations and now weighed about 135. After two days in the sun, I thought I could pull off my charade. I took the added precaution of wearing a knit shirt with wide horizontal stripes in the hope that it would make me look heavier.

That day my mother's sister and brother-in-law were also visiting my parents. I walked into the house and found the group out back on the patio. Everyone greeted me effusively, except for my father, who had great difficulty making even the slightest gesture without experiencing considerable pain. I was immediately taken aback by my father's appearance. He looked hollowed out and all white. His hair was rapidly thinning and the looseness of his clothes testified to how much he had deteriorated. He didn't make a single move without appearing to summon every ounce of strength he had left. He offered me a withered hand that looked like an old branch in winter. I shook the lifeless claw and then let it go. His hand didn't even have the strength to fall, but rather floated back to his lap, where it stayed for the rest of the time I was there.

"How are you feeling, Pop?" I asked.

"Oh, I'm okay, Tony. A little weak, that's all. The pills are supposed to help that."

Suddenly a very strange expression came across his face; he looked at me as if from a great distance and searched my eyes. "How was your trip to Chicago?" he asked.

"Chicago was fine. Very busy. I just got back last week."

"It's good to see you," he said.

We all talked while I stole furtive glances at my father. The tumors in his gastrointestinal tract had caused his lower abdomen to swell obscenely. From time to time, he would rub his temples or forehead in an effort to relieve the pain in his skull.

After a while, my mother and her sister Ann took my father into the house. I asked Ann's husband, Frank, to go for a walk on the beach with me.

It was approaching 5 P.M. and most of the beach crowd had left for dinner. Frank and I walked in silence for a time until I said, "Pop's real sick, Frank."

"Yes, he is, Tony. Is there anything we can do?"

"I don't think so."

We talked about what my mother would do after my father passed away and then I said, "Frank, I want you to know that I have cancer, too. I'm also dying."

Frank stopped dead in the sand and stared at me with a hard expression fixed on his face.

"What did you say?"

"That's right, Frank. Hard to believe, isn't it? I found out last month. I have cancer of the prostate that's spread throughout my body. I've got three years, maybe five. I don't know for sure."

Frank expressed his disbelief and shock. He then asked me about the therapy I was undergoing and I explained the surgery and the estrogens.

"I haven't told Mom, and I don't plan to, at least not now. Not while she has Pop to take care of. She can't have me dying, too."

"Okay, Tony. If that's the way you want it. If there's anything we can do, just tell us."

"Thanks, Frank. I'm sure Mom will need support."

We started back to the house and the rest of the day went smoothly. My mother was so concerned with my father that she barely noticed me. That night I stayed at my house at Long Beach Island and returned to Philadelphia the following day. A week later, my father began having brain seizures. He needed extensive medical attention and we decided to bring him to Methodist Hospital. It was July 30, a hot Sunday. My father was given a private room and heavy dosages of narcotics to relieve his pain. My mother took a room across the hall from my father's. This, of course, presented a problem.

With my mother now living in the hospital, I knew I would have to tell her something about my illness. I could not risk having one of the hospital staff tell her that I had just been a patient here too. After my father was admitted and my mother settled in, she and I went out to dinner.

Both of us were extremely tense. After we ordered our meals, we fidgeted with the silverware, spoke a few clipped and angry words, and then retreated into our own thoughts. Suddenly, we started to argue over whether Pop should have been brought to Methodist weeks before. We snapped at one another like a couple of terriers. Then the tension subsided. I saw the pain in my mother's face. Her large eyes and prominent mouth were turned down in an expression of pity and regret. Her skin was so pale and washed out that even a make-up artist could not have restored the color to it. Finally, the meal came and we began to talk about Pop's condition. Both of us agreed that he wouldn't last long. For a while, we discussed his funeral arrangements.

How should I tell her? I thought. We ate for a few minutes in silence.

"Mom, I want you to know that I have a touch of this, too. But it's okay; we have it under control. I've had some surgery and I'm now getting treatment. I want you to know now before someone at the hospital tells you."

She sat back in her chair for a moment and just looked at me and waited.

"It was local and removed," I lied. "Don't worry. I'm well and now back to work."

"Isn't that what we said about your father's disease? 'Local,' everyone kept saying. 'Don't worry,' they said."

"This is different," I said. I told her that my cancer was in the rib, not in the lung as was my father's, and that the rib had been removed in surgery. "We got it before the cancer spread."

We discussed the situation further and she seemed convinced. She settled down but she no longer had an appetite for her meal.

"Your father knew all the while," my mother said.

"Knew what?"

"Your father knew you had cancer. He told me after we saw you the last time. He said, 'Tony's got it, too.' He just shook his head and kept saying that, 'Tony's got it, too.'"

"Don't worry, I'm recovering," I said. Inside, I was stunned at my father's insight. Suddenly, I remembered that look he gave me. The sick and the dying recognize one another, I thought. I decided to tell him about my disease soon.

The next day my father lapsed into a coma.

On August 6, a Sunday, I went to my office and telephoned Dr. Andrew Von Eschenbach. Dr. Von Eschenbach, an expert on cancer and particularly on cancer of the prostate, is a surgeon in Houston, Texas. We discussed my circumstances at length. When the conversation was concluded I dictated into the tape recorder a memo to myself that would be transcribed Monday. I wanted to record the specifics of our conversation while they were still fresh in my mind, as well as keep a record of my illness.

The memo was dated August 6, 1978. It was addressed to me from me; the subject was "Outlook on Carcinoma of the Prostate in Myself." The memo read as follows:

Following my telephone conversation with Mr. H. Robert Cathcart, President of Pennsylvania Hospital, I telephoned Doctor Von Eschenbach of M. D. Anderson Hospital last week but was unable to reach him. In the interim, Dad was admitted to Methodist and then went into a coma.

On Sunday, August 6, at about 7 P.M., I reached Dr. Von Eschenbach at home.

We had an extensive discussion about carcinoma of the prostate; he is very much interested in the disease because his father recently died from same. He suggested that the orchiectomy be followed by estrogen therapy and hoped sincerely that I would have a good response. Some patients, particularly those in the older age group (fifty years and above) have a remarkable response, but he noted that statistics showing only 20 to 25 percent survival rates up to five years are accurate and stories that people have much higher survival rates are plain myth. He told me that people under fifty years of age like myself have a rather poor outlook and that since I seem to be taking the situation realistically, he might just as well tell me the truth. He suggested that in the event that the estrogen therapy does not work, that I might get x-ray therapy for my back, which would probably relieve the pain but certainly not cure the disease.

He stated that we are talking in terms of 1978 and of course a lot of research is being done and there is always a chance for a breakthrough; nevertheless, my age is against me and a five-year survival would be very exciting but not very likely. I believe he said he had never seen anyone survive five years, at least in my age group. He led me to believe, at least from the tone of his voice, that the future was not very bright.

In addition, there are some chemotherapeutic agents, namely Cytoxan and 5-Fu (chemotherapy), which are being used. Cytoxan appears to have some effect, maybe 30 to 40 percent of patients do have some improvement. He suggested that in the event that I have no response to the estrogens or that the estrogens are helpful for a limited period of time in either providing symptomatic relief or in providing remission, that I then seek the latest chemotherapeutic agents, which may give me some help. He did say that Cis Platinum was being used at Roswell Park Institute in Buffalo (N.Y.). Cis Platinum is a diamino salt which has not yet been released by the Food and Drug Administration and may be helpful.

He stated that in patients who have severe bone pain but no depression of bone marrow that it is their custom to give doses of testosterone, yes, testosterone, which causes the cancer to enlarge. Intravenous dosages of P-32 are then administered. The testosterone sets up the cancer cells for the attack by the P-32. This has been somewhat successful.

He was very cordial and extremely sympathetic and frank and asked how I was responding to the presence of my father in a coma, an overwrought mother, and the realities of a very brief survival. He also suggested that I call him at any time, because there may be moments when a good deal of support is needed.

Conclusion and Summary:

The present course of therapy with orchiectomy and programmed estrogens would appear to be a right direction. In the event that there is no response with the estrogen therapy, as there has not been with the orchiectomy, then perhaps getting into one of the national studies using Cytoxan or 5-Fu would be of some value. It might be of value to write the folks at Roswell Park and see if there would be some potential help in using Cis Platinum or in questioning them about P-32 therapy. In summary, it would appear that the future is not very bright and that I sort out my life, making priorities such that early death is in store unless some dramatic breakthrough occurs. I did discuss with Dr. Von Eschenbach what his advice to patients is, particularly those in my age group with such a dismal outlook, and I think we both agree that continuing "full speed ahead" is the best approach, recognizing full well that life is not always fair.

After finishing the memo, I left my office and went home. My father died the following morning.

I had been busy that morning and planned to go upstairs and sit by his bedside later in the afternoon. Just before lunch, my mother came down to my office and told me that he had finally let go of his burdens. Both of us were relieved that he was no longer suffering. He never emerged from his coma, but died peacefully. He was sixty-nine.

Ann and Frank joined us for lunch, after which they and my mother left together. I went home early that day to think and be alone.

My father's death brought my own mortality into sharper

focus. I suddenly let go of many of the delusions I had been harboring about my own chances of surviving cancer. Over the next few weeks, I set out to put my affairs in order and prepare for death. In addition to my apartment, I owned three other properties—including my house on Long Beach Island and a condominium in Puerto Rico—which I put up for sale. I also sat down with my attorney and rewrote my will to make my mother the sole beneficiary of my estate. After this was completed, I set out to streamline my life by getting rid of many of my personal belongings.

My father's funeral mass was held at St. Francis Church on Long Beach Island in the early evening of August 9. The church was crowded with people, including some priests and nuns who knew my father. My mother was dressed in white, symbolizing the joyfulness of the Resurrection and the opportunity for union with God. Some soft guitar music was played and there were two readings: one by my cousin, a former Roman Catholic priest and now an Anglican priest, and the other by me. My cousin read from Corinthians and I from Reinhold Niebuhr's *Irony of American History*.

"Nothing that is worth doing can be achieved in our lifetime," I read. "Therefore we must be saved by hope. Nothing which is true or beautiful or good makes complete sense in any immediate context of history; therefore we must be saved by faith. Nothing we do, however virtuous, can be accomplished alone; therefore we are saved by love. No virtuous act is quite as virtuous from the standpoint of our friend or foe as it is from our standpoint. Therefore we must be saved by the final form of love which is forgiveness."

The passage was never more meaningful for me than it was that day.

The following day, my father's body was taken in a long procession to the family plot in Hopelawn, New Jersey. It was a hot August day; the air was thick with humidity. The entourage arrived at the cemetery and everyone gathered around the grave site. A priest said some words over the casket and it was lowered into the ground. After the burial, we all went to my cousin Marie's house for the family gathering that customarily follows the funeral. I was there a short while when I told my mother that I had to return to Philadelphia and should be going. I was scheduled to give a presentation before the planning committee of Methodist Hospital's Board of Trustees. We were requesting that $100,000 be set aside to pay for planners to review our building proposal. My mother agreed that I should go and then someone gave me directions to the New Jersey Turnpike, which would take me back to Philadelphia. I got into my rented car and drove off.

I had taken some Percodan earlier in the morning and the pain had not yet returned. The interment, however, had left me depressed and weary.

I drove onto the turnpike entrance and stopped the car momentarily at the booth to get a ticket. Just as I got on the accelerating ramp that joins with the main flow of traffic, I spotted two hitchhikers. They looked as if they were in their early twenties, and I first took them for college students. Both of them had hair down over their ears and were wearing jeans and sports shirts. A rush of prejudice against young people with long hair and wearing what I had come to think of as the uniform of protest—Levi's and sneakers—welled up inside me. I had never had much sympathy for the attacks leveled against the establishment, particularly because it was my own profession that was often being criticized. Now here, suddenly, were two more critics, down on their luck, no doubt, jobless and probably broke, who needed yet another free handout. Coupled with this bias was the standard prejudice almost every American driver has toward hitchhikers. I was well versed too in the horror stories that go with being a Good Samaritan on the American highway.

One might think that all of this was enough to make me

step down hard on the gas pedal and watch these two young men vanish in my rearview mirror. Yet, for reasons I still don't fully understand, I felt compelled to give them a lift. And I have no doubt that I was more surprised than they were when I found myself slowing the car and pulling over to the side of the highway. When the car stopped, I leaned over to the passenger-side door and unlocked it, as the two young men ran up to the car.

One got into the front seat and the other in the back. The young man in the front introduced himself as Sean McLean; the other said his name was Bill Bochbracher. Bochbracher, whom I barely got a glimpse of, was tall and thin and had dark brown hair. As soon as he got into the car, he stretched out on the back seat and apparently went off to sleep. Meanwhile, McLean began to talk with me.

McLean was about five feet seven inches tall, with a muscular build. He had a kind of country freshness in his freckled face, which was accented by a bright smile and a mop of red hair that swept across his forehead and down over his ears.

"What's your name?" he asked me.

"Tony Sattilaro," I said.

"Where ya goin', Tony?"

"Philadelphia."

"We're going to Charlotte, North Carolina. So if you could just drop us at the Philadelphia exit, we'd be grateful."

I said that would be fine. As I drove, McLean said that he and Bochbracher were on their way to Charlotte for a vacation. Both of them had just graduated from a natural foods cooking school given by the Seventh Inn Restaurant in Boston. I asked him a few perfunctory questions and he responded enthusiastically. He went on with some joy about the kinds of foods he was taught to prepare and the importance of cooking for good health. It all sounded very foreign to me and I paid little attention. Still, McLean was good company. He had an innocent, almost naive quality that gave him a certain charm. He seemed free of pretension and filled with a kind of elfish happiness.

Eventually, the conversation got around to me. I told him that I was a doctor and that I had just buried my father, who had died of cancer. "I'm dying of cancer, too," I said. I told him some of the details of my disease and the therapy I had received. He didn't say a word while I spoke. Then, in an almost cavalier fashion, he said to me, "You know, you don't have to die, doc. Cancer isn't all that hard to cure."

I looked at him as if he were just a silly kid. What does a twenty-five-year-old cook know about cancer? I thought. I immediately dismissed what he said as the foolishness of youth.

"Actually, Sean, cancer is very hard to cure. About four hundred thousand Americans die of cancer each year," I informed him. "It's the second leading killer disease in the United States, probably in the Western world. There are no easy answers for cancer, believe me."

"Listen, cancer is the natural result of a bad diet," McLean said. "When you eat lots of red meat, lots of dairy, eggs, refined foods, like sugar and white flour, and foods high in chemical preservatives, then you get cancer. That's if you don't die of a heart attack first. Diet causes cancer," he said confidently. "But you can reverse the disease by changing your diet to one of whole grains and vegetables. People have already done it. And you can do it, too."

I dismissed what he had said as patent nonsense. After twenty years of practicing medicine, I had heard all kinds of quack claims and treated them with the same kind of dignified disinterest that I now showed McLean. I was ready to switch to another subject when he persisted. He wanted to know more about my cancer: How long ago was it discovered? Was I taking chemotherapy? When did the back pain begin? Then he launched off into a monologue on how our daily food gives rise to either health or sickness.

He mentioned a recent government report, *Dietary Goals for the United States,* published by the Senate Select Committee on Nutrition and Human Needs, that he claimed corroborated some of what he was saying. I had never heard of the report. We talked about diet and nutrition all the way to the Philadelphia exit on the turnpike. When we neared the exit, McLean said, "Take us into Philadelphia, okay? Let's go to Essene Natural Foods store. Maybe someone at Essene can help you."

"How are you going to get back to the turnpike?" I asked.

"Don't worry about us," McLean said with a smile, "we'll get a ride."

"Where is Essene?" I asked hesitantly.

"Essene's on South Street. Let's go and see if anyone is there."

If he wants to be dropped at this natural foods store, then fine, I thought. South Street isn't particularly out of my way. I drove to the store and parked.

South Street is a teeming flea market—Philadelphia's answer to the Grand Bazaar. It has always had the reputation of being on the seamy side of the tracks, a home for artists and artisans, wanderers and dropouts. While this is true, there is more to South Street than what its reputation suggests. For some years now, South Street and its surroundings have been undergoing something of a renaissance. Buildings are being rehabilitated; old three-story town houses that were once mere shells have been converted into stylish, even elegant homes. Ironically, much of this has been done by the very young people who during the 1960s probably hung out on the streets here.

Still, one doesn't go to South Street seriously expecting to find a treatment for cancer. But I liked McLean. And if he wanted to be dropped here, I would go along with him.

When we arrived, McLean said, "Let's go in for a minute, Tony. It'll only take a minute."

Essene Natural Foods store was something of an anachronism, a throwback to the days of the old general store. It was a small, narrow store, yet like those old general stores, it seemed to have an inventory the size of a modern supermarket. The store and its contents were far different from any supermarket I'd ever been in, however. It had wooden floors and was softly lighted with natural and artificial lighting. Large barrels contained bulk grains and beans, while wooden crates displayed a wide variety of fresh vegetables and fruit. The shelves were stuffed with all kinds of foods — most of them foreign to my eye — and kitchen equipment.

While I looked around, McLean and Bochbracher spoke to a girl at the cash register. After a few moments, McLean came over to me and said there was no one in the store then who could help me. I had never expected that there would be, but McLean seemed disappointed. I bought some bread and we left. Before we parted, McLean asked me for my address; he wanted to send me some literature on a dietary approach to cancer. I gave him the address and said good-by.

I then went to the hospital and made our presentation to the Board of Trustees. The building program was scheduled to be completed by late 1982; I told the board that I would probably not be around to see the end of the project, but that it was very important to me that it be started. After a short discussion among the board members, the $100,000 we had requested to hire planners was allocated to the project.

That week I quickly got back into the routine of work and forgot about my encounter with McLean and Bochbracher. Later that week, Tony Renzi came into my office and asked me to attend with him a faith healing service given at the Holy Spirit Church, a Catholic church in South Philadelphia. My administrative assistant, Marie Genniro, also urged me to go. By this time I was ready to grasp at straws and agreed to go. The following day, Renzi and I drove to Holy Spirit Church. Marie and her husband Anthony would meet us there. On the way, I became terribly nervous and questioned Tony Renzi at length about what would occur. Renzi explained that there would be a service and a few people would share their experiences with the congregation. Later, we would all pray together. "Don't worry, Tony," Renzi said. "These are normal people who've experienced relief from their illnesses through faith, and they want to share it with others in the hope that they might also get well."

I believed in medicine, not miracles. The chances of a miracle happening to me were so remote that I began to feel hopelessly depressed. I also became disgusted with myself. Next, I'll be turning to the roadside medicine man who sells all-purpose elixir out of the back of a beat-up station wagon, I thought.

Holy Spirit is a modern church, constructed in a semicircle so that the pews radiate out from the altar on an angle, like spokes from a wheel. We sat in the back while a short service was held. Later, a few people got up and gave testimonials crediting God for curing a variety of serious illnesses. There was a short talk about the Charismatic movement within the Catholic church. At the end of the service, those of us who were ill went up to the altar and knelt down. Renzi, Marie and Anthony, as well as a couple of other people who sat near us, went to the altar with me. They all placed their hands over my head and we prayed together.

I was so moved by the love and faith with which they prayed that I could not stop myself from sobbing. After a while, the praying stopped and the service ended.

We gathered outside and I thanked them all for their generosity. A peacefulness seemed to descend upon me. These were good people who had brought me here. They cared, and somehow that made a difference in how I viewed myself and my disease. I had the feeling that I was not dying alone.

By the time I got to my apartment, the back pain was raging again. I went immediately into the kitchen and chased a couple of Percodan tablets down with a glass of water. I slumped onto the couch and waited for the pills to kill the pain. I never expected a miracle, I thought. But I knew I'd go to my grave hoping.

Chapter 4

THE FOLLOWING FRIDAY night, I decided to forget about my troubles by going to Atlantic City. I took a room at a hotel and later went across the street to an Italian restaurant for dinner. Before I went, I took a couple of Percodan tablets, and immediately became concerned about their side effects, which had lately become more acute. Each time I took the pills, I became nauseated, and on several occasions vomited. Now, as I sat in the restaurant eating the pasta, I became increasingly ill. Suddenly, I feared I would not be able to keep the pasta down and abruptly got up from the table, paid the check, and hurried to my hotel. I barely made it to the bathroom before my stomach rejected the pasta wholesale. From that night on, the Percodan had the same insulting effect on my stomach, and I soon had to choose between enduring the pain or vomiting. I tried switching to non-narcotic pain relievers, but found out quickly that they were impotent against the pain. When I went back to the Percodan, the vomiting immediately resumed.

For several days I alternated between pain and vomiting before a friend told me about an acupuncture device that he said might reduce the pain. I had read that acupuncture had been successful in bringing about pain relief and was used in the Orient in place of anesthesia. The theory behind the device was that it stimulated energy to flow along certain pathways, or meridians, which acupuncturists claim exist invisibly just below the surface of the skin. According to some acupuncturists, pain is the result of stagnation along these pathways, which prevents energy from flowing freely along the meridians. This blockage of energy results in pain in a particular area of the body. By increasing the amount of energy flowing into a given area, you unblock the meridian and thereby relieve the pain, or so the theory goes. Between vomiting and experiencing tremendous back pain, I was desperate and willing to try anything. So I bought the device.

It was battery-powered and came with two electrodes that attached themselves to the affected area of the body with the help of suction cups. Each morning I had to attach the electrodes onto the center of my back. After half an hour of contortions and frustration, I managed to get the suction cups attached. However, several times during the day the cups would come unstuck, and I would have to slip into the nearest rest room and try to get them into place again. Not only was this inconvenient, but at times embarrassing. On top of it all, the pain persisted at very nearly the same level of intensity, and it wasn't long before I was back to taking the Percodan and enduring the vomiting. This was an impossible situation. Then I learned about Brompton's Mixture.

Brompton's Mixture is a combination of narcotics: morphine, which kills pain; cocaine, which creates euphoria; and Compazine, which prevents nausea and vomiting. I had read in a professional journal that the concoction was being given to dying patients at hospices. Nearly two weeks after the incident in Atlantic City, I asked our pharmacist at Methodist to make me up a batch.

The day I took my first dose of the Brompton's Mixture, we held a welcome for our nursing students at Methodist Hospital. I was scheduled to give a speech to the new students. Just before I left my office to deliver my talk, I took a tablespoon of the narcotic and then proceeded to the hospital auditorium to address the nurses. As I walked through the wards, I felt the drugs coming on me. I suddenly felt lightheaded and euphoric. There was a new bounce in my walk, and, by the time I arrived at the podium, I was flying. Suddenly, the whole world was filled with wonder. There was no pain, no depression — anywhere. There was only the beautiful earth populated by happy nurses. I gave the best speech of my life. I invoked grand images of new horizons, the high ideals of the medical profession, and the great challenges that awaited our energy and determination. Platitudes and grandiloquence were at my fingertips. I felt like a magician. When my speech was concluded, an explosion of applause shook the auditorium. I was ecstatic. Who would have known I was dying? The Brompton's Mixture was my answer.

It was not without its drawbacks, however. About an hour after taking the medication, my speech became dull and slurred. This usually lasted for an hour, sometimes two. During that time, I saw no one in my office, and Marie Genniro shielded me from telephone calls and visitors. In addition, like the Percodan, the Brompton's Mixture also wore off well before I could safely take another dose to kill the pain. Thus, once again I was left enduring the back pain for several hours each day.

On August 24, I arrived at my apartment with the back pain raging. When I walked into the lobby the security guard on duty gave me a pink postal slip telling me that there was a package waiting for me in the mailroom with sixty-seven cents postage due. I turned around and went to the mailroom and got the package. It was from Sean

McLean. The postage due made sense; it was obvious that these kids didn't have much money, but I was suddenly irritated by the fact that I had to pay postage on a package that I had never requested in the first place.

I went up to my apartment and opened the package. Inside I found a booklet entitled *A Macrobiotic Approach to Cancer.* Macrobiotics? McLean hadn't mentioned the name of the diet. Isn't that the crazy brown rice diet? I wondered. McLean had said that the diet was made up of whole grains and vegetables, but the name was unmistakable. I went into the den and lay uncomfortably on the couch and paged through the booklet.

A Macrobiotic Approach to Cancer was basically a booklet of testimonials given by people who claimed that macrobiotics had cured them of cancer, which in many cases had been diagnosed as terminal by medical doctors. I gave it a rather cursory perusal and was about to toss the thing in the wastebasket when I spotted the name of Dr. Ruth Schaefer, whose testimonial described her successful treatment of breast cancer with macrobiotics. Her statement went on to say that she was a practicing physician in Philadelphia. I put the booklet down and looked up Ruth Schaefer's name in Dorland's *Directory,* the medical directory that lists all practicing doctors in one's local area. I wanted to find out if Ruth Schaefer was really a medical doctor or some fictitious name written into a booklet to give it an authentic ring. I quickly found her name and her home telephone number and decided to call. A man answered the telephone.

"Hello," I said. "Is Dr. Ruth Schaefer in?"

"Do you know my wife?" asked Mr. Schaefer.

"No, I don't. I was just reading a testimonial she gave in the booklet, *A Macrobiotic Approach to Cancer,* and I was wondering if I might speak to her about it."

"I'm sorry," he said. "My wife isn't here. She's in the hospital dying of cancer."

"Oh, I see. Well, you've answered my question. Macrobiotics doesn't cure cancer." I was about to hang up when Mr. Schaefer came back enthusiastically.

"Listen," he said. "It really works. While she was sticking to the diet, it really did help her. She showed real signs of getting well. But she couldn't stick to it. She hated the food."

"Do you think it's worth looking into? I'm dying of cancer," I said.

"Yes, definitely," was Mr. Schaefer's answer.

He then gave me the telephone number of Denny Waxman, the director of the Philadelphia East West Foundation, an educational organization of macrobiotics.

The next telephone call I made was to Waxman. I explained my cancer to him and told him that I had read Ruth Schaefer's testimonial. I then asked him if I could come to see him. We agreed to meet on August 27.

It was raining the night of August 27, and I had some trouble finding the Waxman house, which was located in Bala Cynwyd, an exclusive suburb of Philadelphia on the so-called Main Line. As I drove to Waxman's house, I was filled with trepidation and suspicion. I was certain that I was turning myself over to a bunch of quacks. My mind conjured up all kinds of images of some spurious-looking character dragging all kinds of homemade equipment out of his closet that he would claim cured cancer. I had some deep suspicion of myself, too. I realized that I was desperate and therefore vulnerable. In the end, however, I had no alternative. It was either try something different or die. So I kept driving and looking.

Finally I found the house and was allowed in by a young woman. She asked me to take off my shoes when I entered. I thought this odd, but nevertheless placed my shoes next to the half dozen other pairs near the door. The woman showed me to the study. On the way, we passed a dining room to our left in which five or six people were all sitting on pillows on the floor around a low table, perhaps two feet high. My initial impression was that they were all smoking pot, though I could not smell marijuana. There was a strange aroma in the house, but I guessed its origin to be food. After I had waited a few minutes in the study, Waxman walked in.

I took him to be about thirty years old, five feet nine or ten inches tall. His complexion was bright and slightly tanned. He had an oval-shaped head, with sharp features, narrow eyes, and a long thin nose. The top of his head was bald, except for a few tufts. He was thin, but looked fit. Overall, he had a boyish, even modest quality, but there was a look in his eye of competence and not a little confidence.

He greeted me with a handshake and asked me to describe my condition again. I gave him a thorough description of the cancer, as well as the surgery and the estrogens I was taking. I also showed him the acupuncture device I was wearing on my back. To my surprise, he paid no attention to the device. I had been certain he would make some reference to it, since I doubted that he had any system of his own for treating pain, or cancer for that matter, and would encourage me to use the device. After I finished talking, he began what was for me the strangest examination I had ever received in my life.

The first thing he did was to examine my face thoroughly. Then he looked into my eyes, lifting the lids and asking me to look up, left, right, and down. He then asked me to roll up my shirt sleeves so that he could examine my arms, which he did with painstaking thoroughness. By this time I decided that he was examining my meridians, though what he might have been looking for, I couldn't begin to guess. Next, he asked me to take off my socks so that he could look at my feet. Again, he gave my feet a careful inspection. As he looked at each area of my body, he would occasionally probe a spot on my arms, hands, or feet with his fingertips. This probing was done gently; however, he must have been hitting so-called pressure points because the poking brought about a surprising, indeed inordinate, amount of pain. As he examined me, Waxman didn't say a word. He seemed lost in his own thoughts. Overall, I took him to be somewhat shy, but I was aware of a self-assured and even mysterious quality about him. On top of this, he seemed sincere in what he was doing, so I played along. When the examination was finished, I put my socks back on and we talked for a bit.

"You can be helped," he said to me. "You'll have to eat a strict macrobiotic diet. We'll know if you've got a chance to pull through in three or four weeks."

I searched his face, looking for a sign that might give me some insight into him. Did he have anything? What should I do? In an instant, I decided.

"What is macrobiotics?" I asked him.

"Basically, it's a way of life, incorporating a diet and philosophy to help bring about improved health and happiness. The diet varies some, depending on one's condition, the time of year, and the place one lives. But you should eat fifty to sixty percent whole grains, especially brown rice; twenty-five percent locally grown, cooked vegetables; fifteen percent beans and sea vegetables, and the rest made up of soups and various condiments."

He then told me in greater detail which foods I should be eating. Nearly everything he mentioned was unfamiliar. On the other hand, when he said which foods I should eliminate from my diet, he described my standard fare to the letter. Stop eating all meat, dairy products, refined grains, including white bread and flour products, he said. Cut out all sugar, all oil, nuts, fruits, and carbonated beverages, and foods containing synthetic chemicals and preservatives. He said that the standard macrobiotic diet normally includes some fish, fruit desserts, and other natural sweeteners, but because my condition was so severe I should eat strictly until I showed real signs of improvement.

"My wife is giving a cooking class this Saturday," Waxman said. "Why don't you come to it? This way you can get more advice and become familiar with the foods and the cooking methods."

I left the house feeling a deep sense of confusion and despair. Going there and being given an examination by a thirty-year-old kid who hadn't been to medical school was surely reaching the bottom of the barrel. I had absolutely no faith in this, but something told me to go back on Saturday for the cooking class. I'm not even sure what it was — something in Waxman's manner, the comments made by Ruth Schaefer's husband, and a fundamental confidence in my own judgment. It won't take me long to see if there's anything of value here, I told myself. I decided to find out more about macrobiotics. What did I have to lose?

That Saturday, on Labor Day weekend, I went to the Waxmans' house for the cooking class. There were seven or eight other students there. Most of them were young, but a couple appeared to be in their forties. I looked at their faces; they were eager and enthusiastic and my deep skepticism made me think that these people must be terribly naive. They can afford to be naive, I told myself; none of them is sick. After a while, it became apparent that most of the students were familiar with macrobiotics. We all gathered in the kitchen and waited for Mrs. Waxman to arrive.

Judy Waxman's kitchen was large but typical in design: wooden cabinets, Formica counters, a wooden chopping block, and all the requisite appliances. The kitchen was orderly and neat. What made it different from any other kitchen I had ever been in was the assortment of colorful foods on parade. On every shelf, Mason jars displayed a variety of beans, some red, others black, green, or yellow. Other jars contained what I took to be different grains, most of them dark or golden. Much of the rest of the food — some of it labeled with Oriental characters — was a mystery. On top of one of the counters were several kinds of vegetables: carrots, with the tops still on, onions, leafy green vegetables, which turned out to be kale, and a mysterious long white vegetable that looked like an over-grown, bleached-out carrot. I was told by one of the other students that this was a daikon, a Japanese radish. To one side of the room stood a large bag with the words ORGANICALLY GROWN BROWN RICE printed on it. On top of the stove were a few pots and a pressure cooker.

The kitchen was a stark contrast to my own. I felt my kitchen was well stocked when I had a bottle of wine and some snacks in the cabinet, and some beer and black cherry soda in the refrigerator. Like most busy doctors, I got much of my food on the run, and the great bulk of it came under the heading of "junk food." I couldn't imagine eating macrobiotically.

Judy Waxman entered the kitchen. She greeted everyone with a smile and a slight nod of the head and then proceeded to busy herself for a few moments with the food. As she did, she exchanged some small talk with a few of the students.

She moved around in her kitchen with an almost willowy grace, carrying on conversation while she prepared the food as second nature. Her hair was light brown and pulled back in a ponytail. She had round eyes, set off by high cheek-bones, and a wide, warm smile. She was about five feet five inches tall and had a slender figure. Her voice had a singing quality to it and the trace of an accent, which I guessed to be Eastern European but would later be told was Israeli.

"Today, we'll make a simple meal of miso soup, pressure-cooked brown rice, some lightly boiled vegetables, and a sea vegetable dish of hiziki seaweed and carrots," said Mrs. Waxman.

She then proceeded to the meal. First she poured brown rice into a pot, added water, and stirred the contents gently counterclockwise. The rice and the water were poured into a colander, allowing the dirty water to strain out. This was done three times. The rice was then added to the pressure cooker with several cups of water and a pinch of sea salt. Then the lid was fastened down and the regulator placed on top. She put the rice on a high flame and gave her attention to the vegetables and seaweed. Judy Waxman put the seaweed in an earthenware bowl, poured some water into the bowl, and let the seaweed soak. Then she cut the green tops off the carrots and placed the greens in the refrigerator. "We shouldn't waste any part of a vegetable," she said. "Carrot tops are an excellent and nutritious green. Also, we don't peel the carrots, since so many of the nutrients are at the surface." With that she scrubbed the carrots and daikon with a vegetable brush. The kale was washed by hand. In the meantime, the rice came to pressure and she turned the flame down low. The pressure cooker issued a low hiss for the next forty-five minutes while it remained over the low flame. Meanwhile Judy Waxman gave instructions on the recipes and some of the philosophy behind the macrobiotic diet and cooking methods.

"Our food should be handled with respect and gratitude, because we realize what food means to us. Each day, we are nourished by it; it gives us life; but food is more than simple fuel. It is transformed into our blood and cells. In this way we are recreating ourselves every day with what we eat. If we take food that is fatty, or filled with artificial chemicals, or is chaotically prepared, we soon become sick and chaotic. If we take clean, good-quality food, that's prepared simply and with gratitude, we become healthy, clear-headed, and better able to do whatever it is we want to do in life.

"It's like building a house," Judy Waxman continued. "If

we use bad building materials, the house soon collapses; if we build our houses with strong flexible materials, the house lasts a long time and serves us well."

According to Mrs. Waxman, the macrobiotic philosophy maintained that cooking is the highest art form, since it is the only one that directly changes the blood quality and cells of the body. Although we are moved in one way or another by all art, no other art form more radically transforms our bodies and minds than food and cooking. Thus, one's intention is very important, she said, since the artist-cook can bring about healing or sickness with what he or she creates.

It was at this cooking class that I heard for the first time the words yin and yang. I didn't pay much attention then. I was being bombarded with so much new information that I had reached sensory overload. What I gathered about yin and yang was that the two words were used to describe opposing forces in the universe, one expanding and the other contracting, one systole, the other diastole. According to the macrobiotic view, these two forces of yin and yang were present in all phenomena, constantly attracting and repulsing one another in an effort to harmonize. Yin and yang also existed in food. The way to healthy eating — according to the macrobiotic claim — was to eat a nutritionally sound diet that balanced the two forces of yin and yang. Thus, foods that were at the extreme end of the yang spectrum — such as red meat and salt — or the extreme end of the yin spectrum — such as sugar, alcohol, or drugs — were to be minimized or avoided completely. Whole grains and vegetables, I was told, were in the center of the yin-yang spectrum and thus brought about a more harmonious condition within the body. This balanced condition resulted in a state of health, or so went the macrobiotic claim.

I found it all vaguely interesting but I quickly tuned out. I was more interested in knowing if I could cook and eat the food than in how yin and yang played a part in shaping it.

Still, I had to admit that after ten years of eating this way, Judy and Denny Waxman looked healthy. So did some of the other people at the cooking class who claimed to have been practicing macrobiotics for some time.

After an hour and a half, the meal was ready. Visually, it was beautiful. The rice was spooned out of the pressure cooker and into a dark wooden bowl. The rice was the color of bamboo. Wisps of steam danced above the rice as one of the women brought the bowl into the dining room and placed it on the low table. The boiled vegetables were colorful and not overcooked to the point that they had lost their essential nature — the way I was used to eating them in restaurants. The black seaweed and carrots also provided an interesting color combination, as did the brownish miso soup. Miso soup, I was told, was a fermented soybean-based soup that was rich in enzymes and bacteria, both of which aided in digestion. The soup had some vegetables in the broth, along with wakame seaweed.

I was eager to try the food. I had never been to a meal in which the people placed so much emphasis on the healing power of the food. I was impressed by the simplicity of it, and by the reverence with which the food was treated.

The rest of the meal was brought into the dining room and placed on a low table. We all pulled up pillows and sat down before place settings consisting of chopsticks and a Japanese porcelain spoon. Judy Waxman asked if anyone would like a fork and I accepted her offer. Before we started eating, everyone joined hands and said a silent prayer of thanksgiving.

I sipped some miso soup and found it salty and unappealing. The wakame was distasteful, and I soon put the soup on the side and took some of the other food.

The rice was palatable, though bland. The vegetables were crunchy and tasted good; nevertheless, I had never been a lover of vegetables, and didn't find them terribly exciting. I nearly gagged on the hiziki. Seaweed was not at all easy to get down, I quickly learned, and I ate only a small portion before I gave up on it entirely. I went back to the rice and vegetables and finished eating the small portion I had taken. I thought about going out for a banana split after the meal, and was about to say something like that for humor's sake when everyone began congratulating Judy Waxman on making a wonderful meal. Indeed, the rest of the group seemed to love the food. Everyone took seconds and didn't stop eating for a good forty-five minutes.

"Does this food get easier to eat as you get used to it?" I asked.

Everyone said it did, and several people volunteered stories of how much they were revolted by the macrobiotic food when they first began the diet. After sticking with it a short time, however, these people said they soon found the food delicious. It was hard for me to believe, except that I saw the others thoroughly enjoying it. When everyone was finished, the plates were brought into the kitchen and some of the women began cleaning up. I was about to leave when a woman who had been in the class walked up to me and said, "You're Dr. Sattilaro, aren't you?"

"Yes," I said. "Who are you?"

"I'm Mona Schwartz. I run the East West Center in Florida. I heard about your case from Denny. I just wanted to tell you that you're going to be fine. Don't worry. You're going to get well."

It was the first time in three months that anyone had expressed even the slightest bit of optimism to me, save for the comments made by Denny Waxman. I was visibly moved by her generosity.

"Thank you," I said. "But what makes you say that?"

"I've come a long way, too," Mona Schwartz said. "Someday I'll tell you about my case when we have time. All I wanted to tell you now is that you shouldn't worry.

Just eat the food, be grateful, be active, and think positively. Everything will be fine."

"Thank you," I said again. We then parted and Mona busied herself in the kitchen. I soon left.

When I got out of the house and into my car, I felt as if I had just walked out of another world. What happened back there? I asked myself. I felt as if I had just lived through a dream. I started the car and drove straight to Essene Natural Foods store, owned and run by Denny Waxman and his brother Howard. There I bought $150 worth of food, a pressure cooker, utensils, and a great variety of pots and pans. I piled all of this at the check-out counter and watched as the girl rang it all up. Suddenly a voice from behind me said, "Just starting macrobiotics, eh?" I turned around and saw a young woman.

"Yes," I said. "How do you know?"

"Look at all the stuff you're buying," she said, laughing through her words. "You've got everything there but the kitchen sink."

"Yeah," I said. "And you know, I don't know how to use one single thing in that pile of stuff."

We both had a hearty laugh, which lightened my mood considerably. I suddenly felt that I was on an adventure. Don't take it all so seriously, I told myself as I drove home. It's only food.

When I got home it was still early afternoon so I decided to begin immediately. I planned a simple meal of brown rice, vegetables, and beans. In a short while, I had everything in pots and over a flame. I had washed the rice just as Judy Waxman had and added several cups of water. I put the beans in a big pot of water and turned them on. I cut up some collard greens and onions and placed them in a frying pan. I added some water to the frying pan and began sautéing the mix.

Suddenly, I couldn't remember if I had added salt to the rice and water in the pressure cooker. Is it all that important? I wondered. Should I call Judy Waxman? No, I'll look like an idiot if I call. It'll be all right, I decided. Next time remember the salt!

In order to relieve my anxiety, I went into the living room and put some Cole Porter music on the stereo. I went back into the kitchen and surveyed the pots and pans. It was going to be awhile before the rice and beans were finished, so I decided to turn off the greens and onions for the time being. It was 3 P.M. Two and a half hours later I had finished destroying the meal. The rice was burned black. The beans were hard as little pebbles. I decided the collard greens and onions weren't worth it. I left everything on the stove and slumped onto the couch, depressed and feeling like a fool. I felt an overpowering urge to give up. Macrobiotics is not for me, I thought. I was hungry so I ate some rye bread with tahini nut butter on it that I had bought that day. That was my meal. It wasn't bad tasting. After a while, I started thinking about Judy Waxman's meal. I knew I could eat the rice and vegetables; I could probably eat the miso soup, too. The seaweed was going to take some time.

The next morning I called Denny Waxman and told him that I could not cook the food. Were there any restaurants in town where I could get macrobiotic food? I asked. No, he said. Then he was silent for a moment.

"Let me call you back," Denny said. "I may be able to do something."

Later that day, Waxman called me back and said that it was fine with his wife if I came to their house every day to eat my meals. Judy Waxman would make enough for me to take for lunch the following day. I could make my own breakfast of miso soup and oatmeal. I was overjoyed. Yes, I would take him up on his offer. I told him I would pay for my meals and thanked him for his generosity.

Chapter 5

I WENT TO THE WAXMANS' house that following Tuesday night for dinner. I arrived just before six-thirty, took off my shoes and placed them next to all the others near the door, and walked into the dining room. The five people already present introduced themselves. They were Jerry Moore, Charles Hugus, Scott Moses and his wife Barbara, and Gazina Pollitz. They were all in their middle twenties, except for Gazina, who was in her late thirties. These five people lived with Denny and Judy in this large Tudor-style house. They were all studying macrobiotics under Denny, and all had plans of one day teaching the macrobiotic philosophy in one way or another. The six of us made small talk for a while until Denny walked in and dinner was placed on the table. Each of us pulled up a pillow and sat down at the low table.

I found sitting on the floor irritating and uncivilized. I wondered why they had done away with the chairs. I noted the Japanese porcelain spoon and chopsticks again and wondered if the Waxmans were not adopting the Oriental culture wholesale. I decided not to say anything for the time being; I would wait and observe. The big question remained: Could macrobiotics cure my cancer? If it couldn't, there wouldn't be any point to complaining about the form. I would simply abandon the whole thing.

Just before we began serving ourselves, the little group paused in silent prayer. This was not my custom, but I followed suit. Help me, God, I thought in the silence. Then I opened my eyes and joined the others in taking some food.

Once again I noticed that the meal was very appealing to the eye. This time some of the dishes were familiar to me; those that were not were described by someone at the table.

A small china bowl containing the brackish miso soup was placed in front of each of us. Brown rice, the color of sandalwood, occupied the center of the table in a large wooden bowl. There was an assortment of other dishes surrounding the rice in smaller wooden or earthenware serving bowls. In one of the bowls were collard greens and white Japanese radish, daikon, cut in thin slices; in another was a large serving of the black, stringlike seaweed, called arame; another, larger bowl contained buckwheat noodles, called soba, in dark broth; and in yet another dish were square, white blocks of bean curd, called tofu. The tofu, rich in vegetable protein, is made of soybeans, ground up and formed in squares with a consistency somewhere between pudding and cream cheese. The tofu was garnished with scallions and lightly seasoned with tamari. Tamari, someone pointed out, was soy sauce, but unlike the kind one normally gets in an Oriental restaurant. This was made in the traditional Japanese way of fermenting the soybeans for at least two years without the use of chemicals, preservatives, or sugar. According to macrobiotics, tamari is rich in enzymes and bacteria and reputed to aid digestion. It is moderately high in salt and for this reason I was admonished not to season foods at the table with it.

I took my spoon in hand and began eating the briny-tasting miso soup, along with some vegetables and wakame seaweed that were in the broth. The soup was very foreign to my taste and I found it barely palatable. The wakame seaweed was very distasteful; it was dark and slimy and slithered down my throat as if it were still alive. I finished the soup and moved on to the main meal. With my chopsticks I managed to get some rice and vegetables onto my plate. Despite several efforts, however, I could not manipulate the chopsticks well enough to get the noodles out of the serving bowl.

"Would you like a fork, Dr. Sattilaro?" Judy Waxman asked.

"Mrs. Waxman—" I began.

"Please call me Judy," she said.

"Okay, Judy. Thank you. But no, I won't be needing a fork. From this day forward I'll use chopsticks like everyone else."

With some determination and a few losses, I managed to get some noodles on my plate and into my mouth. They were nearly tasteless. The rice was also understated, if not bland. Nonetheless, it was filling and I ate a good deal of it. The greens and daikon were good, though slightly bitter. The tofu was virtually flavorless, except for the tamari, which could rescue the taste of almost anything, I decided. For this reason I was tempted to drown the meal in the stuff, but Denny was strongly opposed to such a move. He said it would hurt my chances of recovery.

We ate in silence. There was a slight tension in the air that is usually present when a newcomer joins a closely knit group. I sensed that everyone was a bit self-conscious and there were only fragments of conversation, punctuated by an occasional request to pass the rice or vegetables. I had been concentrating on getting the food into my mouth with the chopsticks. I was self-conscious, too, about using the chopsticks awkwardly, but I was determined to master them. So far, I was managing. When I finished my portion of rice and vegetables, I reached with my chopsticks for seconds.

"Use the other end of the chopsticks, please, Dr. Sattilaro," someone said. The voice cracked the silence like a whip. I suddenly felt awkward and on display. Slightly embarrassed, I switched the chopsticks around in my hand and took a smaller portion of the rice than I wanted. The rebuff seemed to make the tension in the room all the more intense. I went back to focusing on my meal. No one spoke for several minutes.

I had not tried the arame seaweed yet, and finally, with some trepidation, I tasted it. Charles Hugus, a handsome young man with short brown hair and playful-looking eyes, broke the silence by asking me how I liked the seaweed. He must have noticed that I had been saving it for last.

"It tastes like unrefined sewage," I said.

Everyone at the table broke into laughter. Charles clapped his hands and laughed out loud. Denny laughed heartily and Judy demurely covered her mouth and laughed, too. The tension suddenly evaporated. When everyone had regained their composure, conversation began and the group relaxed. A couple of people encouraged me to eat some of the seaweed and I managed to get a little down.

"The seaweed will be instrumental in helping you get well," Denny told me. "After a while, you'll even like it. You'll see."

I could not imagine my tastes changing so radically that I would actually like the seaweed. Yet, perhaps Denny and the rest were right; perhaps my palate would change. After all, I thought, I was used to eating fancy foods, covered with heavy sauces and dressings. The food I had lived on for the previous forty-seven years was rich and usually heavily seasoned. Macrobiotic food, on the other hand, was simple and basic, and thus to my palate nearly tasteless. In the case of seaweed, even repugnant. Fortunately, I was never much attached to any particular type of food or ethnic cooking style. I did not live to eat. I enjoyed food, but it was not the center of my life, as it was with many of the people I knew. I was not nearly so attached to my former eating habits as I was to my life. Thus, my dislike for the food was not enough to keep me from experimenting with the diet.

As we finished eating that Tuesday night, I began to ask a few basic questions about macrobiotics. Denny provided most of the answers between mouthfuls. Soon the meal was concluded and I asked the question that most concerned me: "How does macrobiotics treat cancer?"

Denny paused several minutes before he answered. Meanwhile, the table was cleared off and a mild tasting twig tea called bancha, or kukicha, was brought out and placed in front of us. We sipped some tea. Denny's nature, I quickly came to realize, was introverted and shy. Before he spoke, he tended to pause, as if he were reviewing what he was about to say. There was a strength in him, but he seemed somehow removed.

"The dominant view of cancer is that the disease is our enemy," Denny said. "So we immediately cut it out, or bombard it with radiation, or chemicals. We try to eliminate it by destroying it. In the process we end up destroying ourselves. Macrobiotics believes that this approach can't work."

With that, Denny launched off into the macrobiotic approach to cancer. What followed appeared to me a combination of facts, folk wisdom, Oriental philosophy, and leaps of imagination. For the next hour and a half, the disease of cancer — an illness I understood as one of infinite complexity — was reduced to a simple metaphor, one that revolved around the idea of balance. My shallow hope that macrobiotics might have an answer to cancer was reduced in stages, as Denny delved deeper into the macrobiotic approach to disease.

He began with a short history of the American diet, pointing out that since the early part of the century, our diet has steadily degenerated. In 1900, Americans ate mostly whole grains, fresh vegetables, and fruit, with a much smaller proportion of red meat, dairy products, artificial colorings and preservatives. This is not to say that they were not eating meat, eggs, cheese, and other such foods, but that they were eating much less of them than today. The diet was centered around complex carbohydrates, particularly those derived from whole wheat, potatoes, barley, oats, and rice.

With the rise in technology in the twentieth century came the much more synthetic diet that we eat today. Most of our food is heavily processed. The vegetables we eat usually come out of a can or a box. Moreover, vegetables are generally regarded as an accessory to the principal food, which is meat. The modern diet contains little if any whole-grain products. The grains we eat have been refined, which strips them of many vitamins and nutrients, as well as the all-important hull or bran. We have white bread and white rice, and as a result there is very little fiber in today's diet.

On top of this, we tend to eat many of our meals outside the home. As a result, a large portion of our diet is inevitably composed of fast foods, such as hamburgers, hot dogs, and fried and oily foods.

Thus, over the past eighty years, our diet has shifted dramatically from one that was composed chiefly of grains and vegetables to one that is centered on animal products, to the extent that between 40 and 45 percent of our total dietary calories consist of fat, most of it saturated animal fat. Refined grains and packaged vegetables, sugar, and artificial chemicals make up the rest of the regimen.

At the same time that the diet has undergone these dramatic changes, we have witnessed an incredible rise in the incidence of certain degenerative diseases, particularly cardiovascular disease (illnesses of the heart and arteries) and cancer. Denny claimed that the increase in these illnesses is due largely to the degeneration of the American diet. "It's the diet that's killing us," he said.

In countries where a diet similar to macrobiotics is eaten, there is an extremely low incidence of heart disease and cancer, and this has led scientists to believe that cancer and cardiovascular disease could be prevented through proper eating habits.

The scientific evidence linking diet to cancer, heart disease, and other illnesses is mounting and getting a great deal of attention, he said, and he urged me to read the government report *Dietary Goals for the United States.* This, he said, would provide me with an overview of some of the evidence linking diet to illness.

I had real problems accepting Denny's argument. I was not familiar with the evidence he spoke of and I was not willing to concede that diet was the root cause of cancer as well as other diseases. This seemed to be an incredible oversimplification of the etiology of cancer and heart disease. Diet was obviously important to maintaining health, but to suggest that it was directly responsible for bringing about cancer was carrying matters too far. His line of reasoning did not take into account several other possible causes of cancer, including a genetic predisposition, a virus, or carcinogens in the environment. Cancer and cardiovascular disease seemed to me to be distinctly different illnesses, with very little in common except that they both killed the patient.

Moreover, it is no small matter to attack the American diet, long regarded as the best in the world. The United States provides the greatest diversity and quantity of food in the world's history. We are the breadbasket, the horn of plenty. Those few illnesses associated with diet that I was familiar with were due to dietary deficiencies, such as lack of vitamin A in blindness; lack of calcium or vitamin D in rickets; lack of iron in anemia. Yet, these and similar problems were controlled simply by increasing the amount of nutrients in the diet. The consensus was that the problems related to food sprang not from having too much, but rather too little.

The macrobiotic argument was going in precisely the other direction, arguing that — to a point — less was better and that most of us were unknowingly getting too much. Our diet was too rich for the human body to consume and at the same time maintain health. Hearing this for the first time was like being told that the emperor had no clothes. I could not accept it.

While I considered these points, Waxman paused a moment and drank some tea. He set the cup down on the table and then told me that not only did improper diet cause cancer, but, if used properly and in time, correct diet could play an important role in successfully treating the illness as well. Here he introduced me to the fundamental concept of balance in the macrobiotic approach to health and sickness. He made it clear that he was giving me the macrobiotic perspective on treating cancer. He did not claim any scientific evidence supporting such theories, but said that if I stuck with the diet I would experience much of what he was saying.

In order for the body to have any degree of health, there must be an equilibrium maintained between the amount of food coming in and the calories burned in energy and discharged in waste, he said. If we take in more food than we need for energy and replacing cells, the excess is stored in the form of fat. Also, if we eat foods that are difficult to metabolize, such as saturated fat and cholesterol, these foods will also be stored within the body. Much of the excess, of course, is discharged through the urine, bowels, skin — in the form of perspiration — and burned up in activity. But the remainder is stored within the body. Moreover, we are a sedentary people today and thus are unable to burn great amounts of excess in exercise; this adds to the rate of accumulation that goes on.

Denny maintained that for the overwhelming number of people today, this equilibrium was destroyed long ago. We are taking in far more than we can possibly burn up or discharge. As a result, the body suffers under the enormous strain of having to store large quantities of this excess saturated fat, cholesterol, artificial ingredients, and the empty calories from sugar and refined grain products. This accumulation is extremely debilitating because the first thing that happens is that our blood becomes polluted with toxins. These toxins spread to every cell in the body and degeneration begins, initially in the form of fat deposits that collect in the arteries and around the heart.

The disease Waxman was talking about was atherosclerosis, an illness millions of Americans do indeed suffer from. Atherosclerosis is characterized by fat deposits clogging the arteries and surrounding the heart, thus reducing blood flow to the heart and brain. The disease can begin at a very early age. Children under ten have been found with signs of the disease, and autopsy studies performed on soldiers killed in Vietnam showed that these young men were uniformly suffering from clogged arteries; some of them had major arterial closure due to fat deposits blocking the flow of blood. I would later learn that this illness is indeed linked to a diet high in fat.

This accumulation of fat in the body eventually gathers in and around our organs, particularly around organs that cleanse the blood or serve in one way or another to discharge excess, Denny said. Breast lumps in women, for example, are the result of the accumulation of fat, along with certain other toxins in the body, including strong stimulants such as caffeine. These lumps form in the breast because the body is attempting to discharge the excess from the system. When a woman with breast lumps gives birth and breast-feeds, her lumps often disappear. This is also the reason, he claimed, why breast-feeding mothers have a lower incidence of breast tumors than non-breast-feeding mothers. Accumulation, such as this, is occurring throughout the system of those who live on the typical American diet.

Eventually, this accumulation becomes so advanced that cells begin to break down under the stress and we begin to see signs of chronic problems: high blood pressure; heart problems; diabetes or hypoglycemia; loss of sexual vitality; difficulty in urinating; chronic constipation or diarrhea; emphysema or asthma; menstrual problems in women or vaginal discharges. These are signs that the body is under enormous stress and is running down. If a person with one or more of these problems does not change his or her diet, that person is heading for a major disease, said Denny.

To prevent degeneration from taking place throughout the system, the body makes an effort to concentrate the toxins in one or more areas, he said. This is done so that other organs can function properly. When the toxins are concentrated in this way, the result is a tumor and ultimately cancer.

Thus, macrobiotics views cancer and cardiovascular disease and all other degenerative illnesses as one sickness. It is simply a progression of degeneration. At the same time, macrobiotics does not see this disease as somehow apart from the rest of the body, but rather, the disease is the body's response to the toxic environment within the person. This condition, created through unhealthful eating, prevents the body from successfully fighting off other carcinogens in the outside environment, such as contaminants in the air or work place. These trigger the onset of the disease, which was already lying dormant within the body, Denny stated.

What determines the location of the tumor and cancer cells, according to the macrobiotic view, is basically the kinds of foods that gave rise to the disease in the first place.

He contended that although we can generalize about the American diet, the reality is that everyone eats a little differently. Some people eat more steak, others more eggs; some are addicted to sugar, or caffeinated beverages, while others can't stay away from oily, greasy foods. A person who has studied macrobiotics looks at the condition and tries to determine what group of foods gave rise to it in the first place. Then the condition may be treated effectively.

In order to change the condition, Waxman stated, the person must first change his or her attitude toward health and illness. People must recognize that they themselves created the disease and are responsible for reversing it. They must have a positive attitude toward change in order for any healing to take place.

At this point I was confronted with what appeared to be another macrobiotic leap of imagination. Waxman argued that cancer afflicts a person physically, mentally, and spiritually, and thus the disease could not be successfully dealt with unless all levels of the individual were addressed. To do this one needs an all-embracing approach that deals not only with the physical manifestation of the disease but with man's place in the universe.

That approach is based on the philosophy of yin and yang. This philosophy, Waxman said, was developed in China many thousands of years ago; however, it is a philosophy that has also been practiced and understood by many traditional peoples of the West, he said. It is an approach to life that helps mankind understand both the metaphysical and the material phenomena of life. Waxman maintained that by using this concept of yin and yang, one was applying one's highest philosophical judgment to the practical problems of everyday life, including regaining and maintaining health.

"The philosophy of yin and yang is so simple and so profound," Denny said, "but it is foreign to the way

Westerners are used to thinking and at first a little difficult to grasp. So, why don't we go into it at a later date."

For now, you should view cancer as an extreme imbalance in the body, said Denny. In order to restore health, we must reestablish that state of balance. We do this by recognizing what conditions — both nutritional and environmental — gave rise to the extreme condition, and at that point attempt to balance it through the use of food and daily activity. By restoring balance we allow the body to naturally rid itself of the toxic condition, he said, and thus the body heals itself with time. In effect, Waxman was contending that if we reestablished this equilibrium, the body's immune system could recover sufficiently to fight off the disease of cancer.

For a few minutes Denny and I sat there in silence. Questions flew around in my mind like bees around a hive. But I felt it was better not to talk now. I had a sinking feeling inside and I wasn't sure what I was going to do. I needed time to be alone and digest all of this. Perhaps it would look better to me later on, I thought. One question pushed itself to the forefront of my mind and finally I turned to Denny and said, "Whose thoughts are these?"

"Most of them come from a man named Michio Kushi," he said.

"Who is Michio Kushi?"

"He's president of the East West Foundation. He's a philosopher, teacher, and author of several books on Oriental medicine and natural healing. He lives in Boston. Michio Kushi was a student of George Ohsawa's. Ohsawa is actually the man who resurrected macrobiotics from ancient literature and traditions. It was Ohsawa who used the term 'macrobiotics.' Actually, macrobiotics has been practiced on virtually every continent and by nearly every traditional people. They didn't call themselves macrobiotics, of course, but they lived on the food from the land and according to natural laws."

I took a sip of tea. It was cold and had the faintest taste. I thanked Denny for the talk and then left.

That night I wrestled with what I should do about macrobiotics. There was no scientific evidence to support the claim that diet could be instrumental in treating cancer. Even the concept of prevention appeared to me gravely in doubt. In fact, there was little if anything in macrobiotics that stood up to logical scrutiny. Macrobiotics was based on a foreign diet—foreign at least to a Westerner's palate—on daily activity, and on some wholly unquantifiable factors, including faith in the diet's healing capacities and the philosophy of yin and yang, the most inscrutable aspect of all. I cringed under the sound of those words. Were the Waxmans putting me on? I wondered.

The macrobiotic way of diagnosis was also highly suspect. How could one determine which foods gave rise to specific conditions? As far as I was concerned, food, once digested, is broken down into its essential components: carbohydrates, proteins, minerals, and fats. Once it is in this state, it is irrelevant where the protein originated. How could a protein from a bean affect the body differently from a protein from a cow?

Of course, all of this seemed impossible to document, except perhaps the health effects of the diet and exercise upon the body. Even that seemed fraught with difficulty. In the last analysis, macrobiotics was a faith system, and one that I had little faith in.

But how could I have faith? My experience and analytical mind could not accept that these people—most of whom had no medical or scientific training—could have an answer to a problem that baffled the greatest scientific institutions, indeed, the most brilliant minds, in the country. We were spending billions of dollars and using the greatest technology in the world on the problem of cancer, and we still couldn't find an answer. How could I possibly believe that these young people—most of them young enough to be my children—with their ancient diet and concept of yin and yang could solve the riddle of cancer?

But I knew I would go back and eat at the Waxmans'. Why? Because I had no other alternative. That was the biggest incentive of all. I had spent hours pondering the maze of my circumstances and the possible choices available to me, and I kept coming back to the same brick wall over and over again. There was no other place to go. I would not give up the standard treatment I was receiving, but I was forced to try for a long shot. Macrobiotics was the only one that was presented to me.

As long as I regarded it as an alternative, I did not have to take it too seriously, since I basically did not have any faith in alternative cancer treatments, whether they were in Philadelphia or Tijuana. They were all the same to me, and all of them came under the heading of quackery. But when you are dying you become desperate, and your prejudices and pride become luxuries you can no longer afford. I would try for the long shot, I told myself.

That was my rational mind talking. However, deep within, on some emotional level, I found the macrobiotic approach intriguing and even somewhat appealing. It was so far out, so foreign to everything I was familiar with, that I began to think that this was one dark horse I should have another look at.

So every night that September I went back to Denny and Judy's house for dinner. As we had planned, Judy made enough for me to take for lunch the following day and I made my own breakfast of miso soup and oatmeal. I was back at the hospital full-time now. Each day I carried to work my little Japanese lunch box containing brown rice and vegetables. People at the hospital looked at me with a combination of curiosity and pity. There was also a strange disappointment in their eyes, as if I had gone over to the other side. "He's turned himself over to the quacks," many of them must have thought. I would have thought the same thing, had a colleague of mine resorted to macrobiotics in his dying days.

The pain was still with me as great as ever. I was now alternating between the Brompton's Mixture and the Percodan; by using the Percodan less often, my body was better able to deal with the drug and its side effects. I had also gained a tremendous amount of weight as a result of the estrogens. Within weeks after I began the treatments, I went from 140 pounds to 170, much of it water retention. I was bloated and my skin itched profusely. As a distraction, I threw myself into planning our building program and into macrobiotics.

The diet and philosophy were actually becoming exciting for me in the way that any new course of study had been in my past. I became a student again at the Waxman table. I would question Denny thoroughly on the health effects of each food being served and the application of yin and yang to the meal. Everyone else usually joined in answering my questions and asked some of their own as well. Mealtime became almost a study session in a foreign discipline. This became a kind of therapy for me, and usually lightened my mood considerably.

The taste of the food quickly became familiar, though hardly enjoyable. I still found the seaweed repulsive, but I was determined to learn to like it. One night I got the idea of naming the various seaweeds in the hope that humor might help me appreciate their flavor sooner. Thus, it became Nora nori, Katie kombu, Wanda wakame, and Anna arame. Everyone at the table thought this was amusing, particularly when I would ask one of them straight-faced to "pass the Helen hiziki, please."

I was continually being reminded of the importance of chewing my food. In the past, I usually ate while engaged in conversation or in a hurry to make an appointment.

Chewing never mattered very much. However, Denny stressed the importance of chewing in digestion and I was regularly reminded to chew every mouthful between fifty and a hundred times. I was to follow the rule of "drink your food and eat your soup."

My seven dining companions—Denny, Judy, Charles, Scott, Barbara, Jerry, and Gizina—were increasingly becoming friends. I learned from them and drew great hope from watching them. They were young, and more importantly they were healthy. Any qualms I might have had about the safety of the food were quickly put to rest simply by seeing these seven people each day. They were fit. Moreover, they were enthusiastic about what they were doing. They believed in macrobiotics implicitly. Finally, each of them believed beyond any doubt that the food would make me well. The importance of this alone is beyond calculation. I was in the midst of a group of people who believed that if I continued to practice this diet I would be cured of cancer. They never doubted it for a moment, and after a while—in my stronger moments—I even started to believe it, too.

This was not always easy. About two weeks after I started macrobiotics, I developed the symptoms of a cold or flu. I was discharging mucus heavily; I had aches and pains, and sometimes a mild fever. I found this odd because one usually gets the flu in January through March, but not in September. One night at dinner I told Denny that I was coming down with something. His reaction surprised me.

"Congratulations," said Denny. "It's a good sign. You're discharging the cancer."

Waxman and other macrobiotics maintained that when the body was coming back into balance between yin and yang, it often contracted the symptoms of a cold or flu in order to discharge in a quicker and heavier manner the toxins that had been building up over the years. Waxman called colds and flu "sicknesses of adjustment," which were the system's way of getting rid of excess on a periodic basis. He maintained that such illnesses could be beneficial to one's health.

This attitude bewildered me and heightened my skepticism. I was worried that I was actually getting weaker from the malignancy. I was concerned, too, that it was the food that was responsible for quickening my apparently weak state. Perhaps the food is undermining my body's defenses such that the cancer is spreading more rapidly, I thought. How does one keep up his strength on this high-carbohydrate, low-fat, low-protein regimen? In my darker moments, I became afraid that this was the beginning of the end. Maybe I needed a steak dinner to keep my strength up. I was tempted to skip the Waxmans' dinner one night and go out for a sirloin.

Finally, I went to Sheldon Lisker for a check-up. Sheldon found no change in my blood tests. Thus, it did not appear that I was getting any worse on the diet. Perhaps it was just a cold; I didn't believe for a minute that it was some kind of cleansing of the body, as Waxman suggested. I decided to ride the cold out. It lasted several days, perhaps a week, and eventually disappeared. I did feel somewhat lighter and a bit stronger after it had passed. I was not sure why, and I did not question the feeling much.

On September 26, a Tuesday, I woke up at my usual hour of six-thirty. Still slightly asleep, I reached over to the night table for the bottle of Percodan. It was a Pavlovian reaction. Suddenly, I was struck by an overwhelming perception. The back pain was gone. Completely disappeared. At first I was skeptical, so I got out of bed and walked around the apartment, searching my back with my mind. There was no doubt about it; the pain was gone. I didn't know what to make of it. It was a miracle, but how? Why? After nearly two years of suffering with an enormous back pain that only heavy doses of narcotics could put down, I was suddenly free of pain. It was like being released from a straightjacket. In something of a state of disbelief, I took a shower and then dressed and hurried to work. There I called Denny Waxman and told him the news. As I spoke to Denny, I finally began to feel happy.

"Denny, do you really think the diet is responsible for the pain relief?" I asked, almost expecting the pain to return any minute.

"Oh yes, it's the diet, Tony. And it's a great sign. You're doing wonderfully," Denny said. He paused a moment or two and then said, "Tony, I think it's time you met Michio Kushi."

*

At dinner that night, Denny encouraged me to meet Michio Kushi right away, as early as the first week in October, if possible. I told him that I had planned a trip to Italy for the first few weeks of October and wouldn't be back till late in the month. He urged me to cancel the trip. He said that traveling for any length of time in my condition would be unadvisable; I'd have to eat on planes and in hotels and restaurants and this would surely ruin any progress I had made over the previous few weeks. Although I was still unconvinced about the macrobiotic approach—despite the fact that the pain in my back had mysteriously gone away— I realized that Denny was right. Why bother practicing macrobiotics at all if I was not going to give it a real chance? I canceled my trip to Rome.

Within a couple of days, Denny arranged for me to meet Michio Kushi at his home in Boston. Before I was to meet Mr. Kushi, however, I had to attend a meeting for hospital nurses in Glen Cove, Long Island. I had been a consultant for the American Hospital Association for several years and I would be attending this meeting on behalf of the AHA. I arrived in Glen Cove early on October 6 with my bags stuffed with rice balls, courtesy of Judy Waxman and company. Rice balls were brown rice wrapped in nori seaweed — a kelp that came in sheets. In the center of each was a pickled plum that served as a preservative to keep the rice from spoiling. I would be away for two days and would have to eat only the rice balls. In order to keep me from getting hungry and cheating on the diet, Judy Waxman made a basket full of rice balls and admonished me not to touch anything else while I was away.

Chapter 6

AT NOON, THE NURSES' CONFERENCE broke for lunch and I sat with several women at one of the tables. The lunch was typical convention fare: minute steak, instant potatoes, some canned string beans, and carrots glazed in butter. Dessert consisted of some weary apple pie and was served with tea or coffee. While the nurses devoured their food, I placed a couple of rice balls on my plate, slipped my napkin onto my lap, and began eating. Nori seaweed is quite black with emerald green highlights, and as I ate the rice ball—as you would an apple—I noticed the nurses at my table casting suspicious glances my way.

"Doctor, what is that you're eating?" one of my table-mates asked.

"This is a rice ball. This black outer coating is nori seaweed; the rest of the rice ball is composed of brown rice, with a pickled plum, called an umeboshi, in the center. It's quite good; would anyone like one? I've got enough here in my bag to feed all of Glen Cove."

The nurses at the table declined my offer, but the rice balls prompted a barrage of questions. "Why do you eat that thing?" asked one.

And so I told them my story: that I had cancer; that I had had enormous back pain; that I had undergone three operations and been castrated; that I was given little chance of living more than three years; and that I had turned to macrobiotics in the hope that my life might be saved. I realized that it was a long shot, I told them, but I had no other alternative. I was cautiously optimistic, I said. I also told them the back pain had mysteriously disappeared.

As I told my story, they ate their meals with increasing disinterest. For the rest of lunch we discussed the macrobiotic diet and philosophy. Later, after our meeting was concluded, one of the nurses with whom I had eaten lunch came up to me in private and said with earnest sincerity, "Doctor, I've never heard a story like that in my entire life."

Early that afternoon I left the meeting and made my way to La Guardia Airport and caught the Boston shuttle. From there I went by cab to Michio Kushi's house in the adjacent town of Brookline. As I neared my destination, I considered Mr. Kushi.

I had heard a good deal about Michio Kushi at the Waxmans' table. He was regarded as something of a living legend among macrobiotic people. He was born in Japan in 1926 and graduated from Tokyo University with a degree in International Law. Shortly thereafter, he came under the guidance of one George Ohsawa, the man Waxman said had resurrected macrobiotics from ancient literature. In 1949, Kushi left Japan and came to America ostensibly to study government and law at Columbia University in New York. Soon, he began lecturing on macrobiotics as the fundamental means for achieving health and world peace. In the early 1950s he was linking the American diet to cancer and other degenerative diseases. He had trouble finding natural foods in the United States then, so he started a small natural foods business out of his basement. Many of the foods he sold were sent to him from Japan. His wife Aveline named the business Erewhon, after the Samuel Butler novel, a favorite of George Ohsawa. In 1978, Erewhon was grossing more than $13 million a year and was one of the leading distributors and producers of natural foods in the nation. Over the years, Kushi had also established the East West Foundation, a nonprofit educational organization for macrobiotics and for improving the understanding between East and West; *East West Journal,* a national monthly magazine with a circulation of more than 50,000; and several macrobiotic natural foods restaurants, including the Seventh Inn in downtown Boston. Over the years, he and Aveline raised five children.

According to the people at the Waxmans', Kushi had a deep understanding of Oriental medicine. It had been intimated that he was something of a psychic and could diagnose a person's health with a glance. Denny had been a student of Kushi's for the previous ten years, and I was given to believe that there were many thousands of other students throughout the world.

He had written several books on traditional Oriental medicine, including the *Book of Macrobiotics: The Universal Way of Health and Happiness; The Book of Do-In: Exercise for Physical and Spiritual Development;* and *Natural Healing through Macrobiotics.* There were also many smaller works and a quarterly publication of his lectures, called the *Order of the Universe.* All of this combined had given him a small empire.

I had purchased a couple of his books and skimmed over them. I was not impressed. It appeared to me that they contained the wildest claims without the slightest bit of scientific documentation to back them up. On top of that, his ideas had something of a mystical ring to them, and much of his teachings seemed based on a foreign tradition and view of the world.

Still, I was eager to meet the man who was the leading teacher of macrobiotics. For me, this was the acid test. Michio Kushi was the source of much of macrobiotics, and if he turned out to be less than genuine, I had decided to break with the regimen.

The cab rounded through the streets of Brookline and finally we arrived at the house. I was immediately taken aback. This was no ordinary house but a Tudor mansion, made of dark brown brick, with a stone portico before the front door and a terrace that overlooked the front of the house. The cab pulled into the drive and stopped beneath the portico. I got out, paid the driver, and walked up the steps to the front door.

I would later learn that the Kushis had bought the house with the intention of converting it into a school for macrobiotics; however, the neighbors were opposed to such a move and this was enough to stop the Kushis. Michio and Aveline chose to live in the house instead and provide room and board for many of their students. However, as I stood there at the door and rang the bell on this October afternoon, I was aware of none of this. Standing there looking into the glass window, I became anxious about what I had gotten myself into in coming here. The thought crossed my mind that Michio Kushi must be the Henry Ford of natural foods. That image did not hold any great appeal for me.

A young woman came to the door and let me in. I took my shoes off, placed them next to the others near the door, and entered a large foyer. To the right was a wide wooden staircase. Beyond the staircase to the right were a couple of doorways. Against the long wall to the left were two doors spaced well apart, which opened up to a living room and an adjoining library. I went into the library and saw Denny Waxman and another young man, who introduced himself as Michael Rossoff. Rossoff was the director of the Washington, D.C., East West Foundation. He was about thirty-two years old, with a slight build, dark features, and a mustache. The three of us sat down on a couch and made small talk for a few minutes. Meanwhile, I scanned the living room and library for insights into the character of Michio Kushi.

The walls of the large rooms were off-white and trimmed in dark mahogany. There were works of Oriental art and others of Occidental origin—all tasteful and appearing to be originals. The Western paintings were nature scenes in colorful oils. There were a couple of Japanese watercolors and a long narrow wall hanging on which only large Oriental characters were painted. Two of the walls of the library were lined with books in English, French, and what I presumed to be Japanese. The English-language titles ranged from classical literature to science to religion to metaphysics. Two Oriental rugs stretched across the floor of the library and living room.

In the far wall of the living room was a large fireplace, out of which jutted a wood-burning stove. The stove seemed incongruous in the midst of such a house. To the right of the fireplace was what I took to be the largest and most beautiful dollhouse I had ever seen. I got up to have a better look at it. At first glance it seemed simple and delicate, but on closer inspection, I realized that it was full of intricate details and exquisite in its workmanship. The dollhouse was a castle made of yellow wood with an ornate, red-shingled tile roof. It stood on a table and from the base to its peak was about three and a half to four feet high. A couple of pennants were draped from small wooden arrows that stood near the gold front doors of the castle. Two small bowls of rice were set out before the doors. Here and there were red, silver, and gold colors.

"What is that?" I asked Denny.

"That's Michio and Aveline's shrine to their ancestors," Denny said.

I looked at the castle again. It was beautiful.

In another room beyond the library I heard a few youthful voices talking. Meanwhile, Michael and Denny talked while I tried to assess what I had seen. Here was a man who had achieved great success; had good taste in art; had a wide view of literature, the sciences, and religion; paid homage to his ancestors; and was concerned about his heating bills. Or was it rather that he was concerned about conserving oil?

Suddenly, from the far door that opened into the library entered Michio Kushi. Before he was within ten feet of us, he was saying, "Hello. Hello. How are you?" He then walked up to me, smiling, and shook my hand. "I'm very pleased to meet you, Dr. Sattilaro."

"I'm pleased to meet you, Mr. Kushi," I said.

"Please call me Michio. No one calls me Mr. Kushi," he said.

He gestured toward the small alcove off the library. The alcove was enclosed by French doors that were draped by long white curtains, and was bathed in the four o'clock sun.

"Please," Michio said. "Let us sit there."

We all entered the alcove and sat down and talked. Now I got a closer look at him. I had noticed when he entered the room that he was tall for a Japanese. He was five feet nine or ten inches, with a slender, wiry build. His hair was jet black and combed straight back, revealing a prominent, sloping forehead. He had small, soft eyes, a flat, wide nose, and a small mouth. He had large, thick ears that stuck out slightly from the sides of his head. He wore a three-piece, dark blue suit, a white shirt, and a tie with a silver and navy print. He spoke with an accent peculiar to Japanese, pronouncing my name as "Sattiraro," and he seemed pleased when I asked him to call me Tony. There was a playfulness in his manner and he smiled and laughed often. His eyes were so soft that I could not decide whether there was some deep sadness there or a happiness akin to bliss. Finally, he asked me to describe my disease. As I did, he listened and watched me intently.

When I finished telling him the medical details, he performed the same examination of me that Waxman had done a month earlier. He looked into my eyes, examined my face carefully, and inspected my arms and hands. He asked me to remove my socks, and then looked closely at my feet. Meanwhile, Waxman and Rossoff looked on with interest.

I felt utterly at the mercy of these people. I had a mounting sense of anxiety. I was used to being in control of such situations. When my doctor performed an examination, I was intimately aware of every step he took; I knew what he was looking for and what he might find. However, as Kushi performed his Oriental diagnosis on me, I was totally in the dark about his methods and what he would say after he formed an opinion. Once again I was reminded of how a patient feels while undergoing an examination by a physician.

Still, Kushi had a reassuring manner. It was obvious that he had great confidence in his methods and he seemed to know what he was looking for. Occasionally, he would probe various points on my body that seemed abnormally sensitive. As he did, he sometimes issued a low growl from the back of his throat. When he had finished, he looked at my face again, this time as if from far away.

"It's not so bad," he said, smiling and shaking his head reassuringly. "Everything will be fine. You must follow the standard diet, but all fish—out! All flour products—out! All fruit, all oil—out! You should wear no synthetic clothing against your skin. All cotton clothes, please. Follow this way, and perhaps in six months all will be well. Really. Problem is not so serious. Okay?" With that he gave me a warm smile. All four of us sat down again.

"Have you seen anyone with this type of cancer cured before?" I asked him.

"Yes, many people with cancer have been made well again through macrobiotics," he said. "Not just cancer, but many other diseases, too. Many people, like yourself, come to me when they have tried everything else with no success.

Macrobiotics is their last resort. Many thousands of people are leading much happier, healthier lives by following the macrobiotic way of life. Macrobiotics has spread throughout the United States, Canada, Mexico, South America, Europe, and Japan. Even macrobiotic communities now in India and Australia."

"I read the case histories. It's too bad about Ruth Schaefer."

"Yes," Michio said. "I feel very sorry."

A young woman came into the room. "Can you give us some tea?" Michio asked. In a few moments the girl returned with four cups of bancha tea. As we sipped the hot tea we continued talking. Michio seemed as curious about me as I was about him. I asked benign questions and listened intently. His speech and manner were simple and direct. I had expected someone quite the opposite of the man who was sitting across from me. Actually, I wasn't sure what to expect, but in my more skeptical moments I had envisioned someone along the lines of a used car salesman with a fast pitch. This was not Michio Kushi; he was confident, yet genuine, even humble. These characteristics, coupled with the fact that he was obviously successful, gave credibility to an otherwise unbelievable claim. Now all I had to do was convince myself that these people weren't incredibly naive or misdirected, living under some pretty-sounding delusion.

Soon someone called a cab for me. Denny said he would escort me back to my hotel. When the cab arrived, Michio saw me to the door.

"Don't worry," he said to me. "Your mother is very strong. She gave you a very strong constitution."

I thanked him and then Denny and I left. As we drove to the hotel, I asked Denny if he had ever said anything to Michio about my parents. Denny said he hadn't.

That night in my hotel room, I thought about Michio Kushi. I didn't know whether he was right or wrong about my condition, but I sensed there was substance and strength in the man. I kept hoping that these people had something, but always some part of my mind refused to believe.

Just before I went to sleep that night, I recalled Michio's comment: "Your mother is very strong." I wondered how he knew.

*

A few days after I returned to Philadelphia, Denny invited me to attend the macrobiotic classes he was teaching at the East West Foundation, which then was located on the second floor of Essene Natural Foods store on South Street. The classes were held Friday nights, and were preceded by an open house dinner. I attended my first macrobiotic class that Friday night.

The second floor of Essene is small for a classroom, perhaps thirty feet by fifteen feet. There were some benches and chairs along the walls, but most of the students sat on the floor. A portable blackboard stood at the front of the room, just before the large windows that looked out onto South Street. The meal, which was served buffet style in large bowls, consisted of brown rice, azuki beans, sliced carrots in hiziki seaweed, and leafy green vegetables topped with a dressing made of umeboshi plums, water, and scallions. Dessert was fruit kanten, which is a gelatin made of fruit and fruit juice, thickened with agar-agar, a powdered seaweed. I passed the dessert but I ate too large a portion of the rest of the food.

That was my failing in macrobiotics. Although I never went off the diet prescribed by Michio Kushi and Denny Waxman, I occasionally overate, particularly when I had a craving for something. I almost never ate a macrobiotic dessert; when I craved something sweet, I would often eat butternut squash or acorn squash, either of which I found delicious and—after I had eaten enough of it—generally satisfying.

There were fifteen to twenty people attending the class. Most of them were young, though a few were of my own age group. Outside of the people from the Waxman house, I knew no one at the lecture.

Soon Denny arrived and waited in the back of the classroom while people finished eating. When the meal was completed and the food removed, he went to the front of the classroom and stood beside the blackboard. Under his arm he held the *Book of Macrobiotics,* by Michio Kushi. He knelt down on the floor and placed the book next to him, then he sat for a few minutes to let people take their places for the class. I observed him as he sat there waiting. There was a strange incongruity in his manner that made him appear shy and yet confident at the same time. He always appeared outwardly friendly, but there was something aloof about him.

"Before we begin tonight's lecture," Denny said, "let's harmonize our vibrations by chanting the sound of su. Let's chant su three times."

With that, he asked everyone to sit up straight and breathe deeply. "Now, raise your arms straight above your heads, look up at the ceiling, look straight ahead of you, and now lower your arms to your sides. Place your hands in your laps. Relax. Let's repeat the same motion: arms straight up, look up, look straight ahead, bring your arms down to your sides, and place your hands in your lap. Again, let's do the same motion, please...

"All right, let's sit up straight, place your hands in your laps, palms upward, right hand under the left, thumbs lightly touching. Let's close our eyes and take a deep breath. Inhale deeply...Exhale...Inhale...Exhale...Inhale... Exhale...Now, on the out-breath, this time, let's chant the sound of su three times. Inhale...

"Sssssssuuuuuuu..."

When the chanting began, I couldn't help opening my eyes to look around me. Everyone's face was expressionless.

The whole room seemed locked in a trance. I was familiar with Gregorian chant, and recognized that there was a spiritual basis for chanting, which in essence is simply another form of group prayer. However, chanting always struck me as foreign and somehow mystical, and I was afraid that I was now getting into the hidden, darker regions of macrobiotics. Was this some kind of strange religion or cult? Was chanting the first step toward indoctrination in the group mind? I felt deeply uncomfortable with the whole thing and had to suppress the urge to leave the room.

Soon, everyone finished chanting and for several moments there was silence. Finally, Denny broke the silence by saying in a soothing voice, "Let's sit quietly for another minute and then open our eyes." After a couple of moments, people began opening their eyes and shifting about. Life returned to the room, and Denny stood up to begin the lecture.

That night Denny lectured on yin and yang, the fundamental principle of macrobiotics. He pronounced the words somewhat differently from the way they are spelled; it was yeen and yong, rather than yin and yang. In any event, yin and yang are viewed as the two primordial forces that drive the universe; each has specific characteristics that complement, and at the same time are antagonistic to one another. Yin is the force that brings about all expansion, diffusion, and separation, while yang results in contraction, fusion, and assimilation. Yin and yang are polar opposites, and as such are continually attracting one another to result in unique combinations and an infinite number of forms. Excess yin, or expansion, is constantly attracting a proportionate degree of yang, or contraction, in order to create a balanced condition, or harmony. The macrobiotic view is that the universe is constantly seeking harmony between two opposing forces. Thus, whatever is hot, or yang, will eventually turn into its complementary opposite, which is cold, or yin, to reach a mean temperature which will be a state of balance, or rest. Day turns into night, and back again; the seasons progress according to a cycle of yin and yang—from winter, which is yin, to summer, which is yang. Whatever is high will become low, and the low will become high. This polarity of opposites is further seen in the differences and attraction between male and female, north and south, East and West, plus and minus. This attraction of opposites results in movement, which in turn results in change, thus yin and yang govern all change in the physical universe. According to macrobiotics, yin and yang are observable and can be studied, and, as a result, change is predictable.

Yin and yang are as relevant to the motions of the planets, Denny said, as they are to the food we eat. At this point, he launched into a discussion on the yin and yang of food.

All food has yin and yang influences on the body, he said. That is, some foods create contraction and ultimately tension, while others create expansion and, at the extreme, lethargy and diffusion. Food can be placed on a spectrum from yin to yang, depending upon what effects the particular food has upon the body. At the extreme yin end of the spectrum are drugs, alcohol, refined sugar, and certain dairy products. At the yang end of the spectrum are salt, eggs, meat, and hard, fatty cheeses.

Lifestyles can also be thought of in terms of yin and yang. A more passive, inactive lifestyle is regarded as more yin, while a more physically active, aggressive lifestyle is more yang. In general, yang characteristics are relatively more aggressive, harder, smaller, shorter, and more physically oriented, while yin characteristics are relatively more passive, softer, larger, taller, and more mentally oriented. The more healthy kinds of lifestyle, according to the macrobiotic view, are those that maintain a balance between mental and physical activity. This balance between yin and yang is the essence of a healthy, stable condition.

Denny then went on to discuss the macrobiotic approach to cancer. He repeated pretty much the same information he had given me a few weeks earlier on how cancer and other diseases originate. Once again, it was essentially the idea that disease originates from the accumulation of excessive amounts of harmful foods. In the case of cancer, this accumulation continues until the body begins to store the excess in various places, where ultimately a tumor is formed. The type of cancer and its location depend upon the kinds of foods eaten. Cancer is thus seen as an extreme imbalance of the system of yin and yang. However, while the overall condition might have been brought about by a certain group of foods, it is the opposite type of food that triggers the growth of the malignancy, Denny stated. That is, when the toxic condition in the body is caused by the predominance of overly yang foods, it is the smaller quantity of yin that triggers the malignancy. The same is true of an overall yin toxic condition; it is the yang agent that sets the cancer in motion. Every stick of dynamite needs a spark to set it off. This is yin and yang at work. Cancer is no different.

Denny explained that, in general, cancer caused by yin factors tends to manifest itself at the peripheries of the body, as in the case of skin cancer, and in the hollow, more expanded organs. Cancers caused by yang foods usually are located in the deeper, more dense organs of the body.

In order to treat both types of cancer, the body must be brought back into a state of balance, he continued. Whole grains are balanced between yin and yang. Vegetables are also located near the center of the spectrum, though they lean slightly toward the yin end. By eating a diet centered on whole grains and vegetables, one is rejuvenating the body in several ways, according to the macrobiotic view: reestablishing a balanced condition, eliminating the abundance of such harmful constituents as fat, cholesterol, artificial ingredients, and refined empty calories; and restoring the body's strength so that it can purge the toxins from the system.

Thus, gradually, according to the macrobiotic claim, this process of accumulation begins to reverse itself. The blood and lymph no longer carry these harmful constituents to the organs each day, but are now free to carry such toxins *out* of the body. Further, the organs are no longer overworked by a new arrival of toxic waste each day. As the excess slowly begins to disappear, the body experiences increased vitality and begins to purge itself of the cancer. In order to speed up the process, one needs to be physically active; the person should seek out some form of exercise that he or she feels comfortable doing so that it can be maintained each day, Denny advised. Over several months, perhaps a year, the cancer comes under control and is ultimately eliminated from the system.

At this point I broke in to ask a question. "You're telling me that if I continue to eat this way my body will eliminate the cancer on its own?"

"Your body is not doing it on its own, really," he said. "It is the totality of many factors at work. The food brings the condition back into balance between yin and yang, and it is also making you physically stronger. Exercise and positive attitude are also very important for the person to get well."

"How do you arrive at the idea that whole grains are balanced between yin and yang?" I asked.

Denny's answer was as mystical as the question. He argued that if one were to divide all food into yin and yang, we would quickly see that animals are more yang and vegetables more yin. Animals are more active, aggressive, heavier, and more dense than plants. Vegetables, on the other hand, are expansive, stationary, lighter, and more fragile. Whole grains are the most contracted, hardest, and least fragile foods within the vegetable kingdom. They are more yang than any other vegetables but more yin than animal foods. As a result, they are located more toward the center of the spectrum, he said.

However, there are other reasons why whole grains are

regarded as the principal foods for mankind, he said. An illuminating clue into how we should be eating, Denny said, can be found by examining our teeth.

By natural selection, humankind has evolved so that its teeth are the kind best suited for its survival upon the planet during the present time, said Denny. We have thirty-two teeth: twenty molars and premolars, eight incisors, and four canine teeth. The molars and premolars are best suited for grinding, not tearing. Whole grains are foods that require grinding. "We find it very difficult to chew meat effectively with these teeth, as I'm sure you've already noted in your own life," Denny said. The second type of teeth is incisors, which suggest the cutting or biting off of vegetables. The smallest number of teeth, the canine, which are similar to those of carnivorous animals, are used for tearing animal foods. The ratio of grinding to cutting to tearing teeth is 5:2:1. This suggests that man's principal food should be whole grains; the second food should be vegetables; the third, animal foods. He then went even further and said that if we combine the grains and vegetables, we get a ratio of 7:1; our diet should be made up of seven parts vegetable quality to one part animal quality.

The proof that a diet of whole grains and vegetables is best suited for humans is in the body's reaction to the food. Digestion is smooth and intestinal problems tend to come under control when we eat more fibrous foods, such as whole grains and fresh vegetables.

At this point, Denny took this ratio of 7:1 a step further. When humans reach adulthood, they require fewer calories for rebuilding muscle and bone tissue than for providing energy; their greatest need is for energy. Macrobiotics claims that the ratio of food for energy versus food for rebuilding body tissue should be approximately 7:1. Carbohydrates are converted by the body into calories for energy. Protein, and sometimes fat, are used for rebuilding body tissue. Therefore, the food best suited for our bodies should be seven parts carbohydrate to one part combined protein and fat. The single food that best reproduces this ratio is whole grains, particularly brown rice. Obviously, we can't eat only brown rice, Denny said, so we make the grain the principal food, and complement it with fresh vegetables, beans, sea vegetables, and various fermented products, such as miso, tamari, shoyu, tempeh, and others.

He mentioned other reasons that whole grains are the most appropriate food for mankind today, not the least of which is to provide an answer to the problem of world hunger. By switching to a grain-based diet, he maintained that we could feed the world. "Whole grains will grow almost anywhere, and they have been the primary food for nearly every traditional civilization. They are the primary food for most of the people of the world today." Apart from the health considerations, we have to be concerned about the fact that all over the world people are starving while we feed great portions of our grain harvest to livestock. The only way we can stave off world hunger is to switch from a meat-centered diet to one based on whole grains and vegetables.

"On every level — from individual health concerns to the welfare of the world — the typical American diet is completely out of step with the times, out of balance with the Order of the Universe," said Denny.

With that, the lecture ended and I left.

As I walked from Essene to my car, I was once again thrown into the turmoil of having to deal intellectually with macrobiotics. My initial impulse was to abandon the whole thing that night. It all seemed preposterous to me. As a medical doctor, I could not fit anything about macrobiotics into the frameworks established by my Western medical training. I was continually groping to find the common thread between my own understanding of medicine and the theories presented by macrobiotics. There *was* no common thread, it seemed. As a result, my initial impulse was to dismiss macrobiotics as ridiculous.

What made it worse was the way in which the macrobiotic people reached their conclusions. Virtually every one of the macrobiotic theories had been arrived at by way of some mystical or philosophical interpretation of the universe. They claimed that human intuition and the practices of traditional peoples were their guides. As far as I was concerned, intuition was another word for guessing. Some of their theories seemed absolutely far-fetched: yin and yang; seven-to-one ratios; the healing powers of a grain and vegetable diet; the notion of excess and discharge. If only the world were so poetic as they made it sound, I thought.

Where was the proof for such claims? I kept asking myself. That question came back to me. I had been feeling better since I started the diet. The pain was gone; I was also experiencing a feeling of lightness and energy. Of course, it was too soon to say with any certainty that these symptoms were the result of the diet. But I was beginning to wonder.

There was nothing in my training or my experience to help me deal with the mystical or philosophical aspects of macrobiotics. The East was used to working with intuition, metaphors, and parables; the West relied upon science. I could not bring the two together yet, so I was forced to put aside my criticisms of macrobiotics and concentrate on the few things that I could make sense of. I was feeling better; this was the bottom line for now. I had to focus on the larger question: Would this diet make me well? If it did, then perhaps we could do some scientific studies later to determine how the diet worked. My experience might prove of great value to mankind. If macrobiotics proved to be worthless, then I was no worse off.

Thus, I decided to continue with macrobiotics and hope that I could unravel the metaphorical and philosophical system that had been worked out. I thought of myself as a pioneer or, in my less romantic moments, as a guinea pig.

Chapter 7

IN EARLY NOVEMBER my spirits fell with the leaves. I
was more isolated now than in any other time in my life. I
had two strikes against me: I had cancer and was practicing
macrobiotics. The cancer alone was enough to make people
uncomfortable around me. They were either incredibly
solicitous or so distant that it made me wonder if they didn't
believe cancer was infectious.

I did not make it easy on people. When someone came
into my office and asked me how I was, I sometimes
launched off into the grim details of my illness, the surgery,
and my poor prognosis. I would often take out my x-rays
and go over them in detail with my guest. There was not
much anyone could say.

One afternoon, John Mcellhenny, the vice chairman of
our Board of Trustees, stopped by my office while I was
considering my funeral plans. I turned to him and said,
"John, I wonder if you would do me a favor?"

"Of course, Tony, what is it?"

"I'm planning the details of my funeral now and I'd like
you to be in it. Would you do that, John?"

John and I had been friends for more than a decade and it

took him a few moments before he finally drew a deep breath and said, "Of course, Tony. But isn't it a bit early to be talking about this?"

"I don't think so, John. We know what the data say. It's not good, that's for sure. I think it's best to be prepared."

I sometimes talked excessively about death. In late October, I attended an American Hospital Association meeting, after which I spoke to several other physicians about my illness. There were some pretty frank words exchanged about chances of surviving for very long. None of the doctors thought my chances were good. When the discussion slowly ground to a depressed halt, I began to lecture about the stages of dying, and how our society really neglects the terminally ill. It was clearly a monologue and one that made everyone present extremely uncomfortable. Later I learned that I would not be appointed to another consultantship at the AHA. I telephoned a friend to ask why.

"Well, you know, Tony, if you hadn't been so outspoken about your own death, I think you would have gotten another appointment," the friend said. "I think you really put people off." It would be a full year before I would be reinstated.

By the beginning of November, people were steering clear of me. One day I was walking down Chestnut Street in Philadelphia and spotted an acquaintance walking toward me from farther down the block. The man spotted me and I waved and he crossed to the other side of the street.

Macrobiotics only complicated the matter. I no longer went out to dinner with friends and colleagues. I had also stopped eating my meals at the Union League. As a result, I saw almost no one socially. When I had to attend a professional affair where food was being served, I brought my own. While everyone else was cutting into his filet mignon, I'd be opening my Japanese lunch box and removing a rice ball and some vegetables. This, of course, only served to make me more conspicuous. Most of my colleagues did not care what my eating habits were and regarded me with patronizing curiosity: "Gee, Tony, that's interesting." Others, however, observed a tense and dignified distance; they simply didn't speak to me.

Of course, I understood their feelings. Generally, physicians regard alternative health approaches as charlatanism and a fraud against the public. By indulging in an alternative approach myself, I was seen as lending credence to a system that could be dangerous to other patients.

Nevertheless, by mid-November I was convinced that this crazy diet was making me feel better physically than I had felt in years. For the previous twenty years I had suffered from chronic intestinal problems, particularly regular diarrhea. I had been taking a variety of medications, all of which proved virtually useless. However, within weeks after I began the macrobiotic diet, my digestive problems disappeared. On top of that, I had great reserves of energy and my mind seemed clearer than usual. At first I attributed my increased vitality and mental clarity to my recovery from surgery. However, as time wore on and I continued to feel improvement, I decided that the diet was at least partly responsible; I did not remember feeling this well before the surgery — or before the back pain, for that matter.

At the same time, I was beginning to see some consistency in the macrobiotic use of yin and yang. Every night at dinner, my tablemates discussed people, health conditions, and situations in terms of yin and yang. And after a while, this mysterious and foreign language began to unravel itself.

Ironically, as I gained more strength, I began to feel trapped by macrobiotics. It was clear that if I had any chance of getting well by this approach, I would have to eat nothing but macrobiotic food. This meant cutting off many of the ties of my former life and creating new and even stronger ones with the macrobiotic community.

I did not relish the thought of doing so. The cultural differences between me and the macrobiotic people — at least those whom I had met so far — were enormous. In many respects, I was a paragon of Western values. The macrobiotic people, on the other hand, valued things Eastern. They sat on the floor, ate with chopsticks, and chanted before gatherings. In many cases they lived communally, sometimes as many as ten or more people living in the same house. They were young and healthy, and I was middle-aged and dying. We were not what you would call a perfect match. This was especially true of our temperaments.

I was clearly more yang in many respects than most macrobiotic people I had met. I was ambitious and aggressive in my work. I lived on a tight schedule and tried to take advantage of every minute of the work day. The macrobiotic people, on the other hand, generally maintained a casual approach to life and, compared to me, seemed unambitious. Meetings and lectures rarely started on time, and when they did they usually dragged on interminably. Denny's lectures were loosely structured and usually ran on for two and a half to three hours a night. On top of this, no one that I had seen lecture had been trained in public speaking. The lectures often lacked punch and entertainment.

I eventually persuaded Denny to start the classes and meetings on time, and to cut his lectures to an hour or an hour and a half. Because of my many years of experience as a public speaker, a medical-school teacher, and a graduate of Dale Carnegie, Denny was willing to listen to me, and as a result he improved his presentation and delivery.

Still, I was continually attempting to separate the form of macrobiotics, or the way it was practiced, from the substance, which to me was the therapeutic effect of the diet. This was not always easy.

When the weather turned cold in early November, I discovered that the macrobiotic people did not believe in keeping their houses warm in the winter. Temperatures inside the house usually hovered between sixty and sixty-four. Sometimes the temperature would drop into the fifties. One night, while we were having dinner, I took a deep breath and exhaled and noticed that I could see my breath.

"Denny, look! For God's sake, I can see my breath. Why don't you people heat the house? We'll freeze to death by January if this keeps up."

Denny laughed good-naturedly. "I think we'll make it through the winter, Tony," he said. He then proceeded to tell me why they kept the house cold. In order to live in accordance with the season, he said, people should respond to the winter as nature does. In winter nature contracts. Everything goes inward. The sap of the tree goes deep within its trunk and roots. The leaves fall off the trees. Water turns to ice; rain turns to snow. The ground becomes hard and dense. In order to adapt to the season, we must do the same thing. To do that, he said, macrobiotic people cook for longer periods of time—cooked food is more yang—do more baking and more pressure-cooking. People living in more temperate climates should not eat foods that are from tropical or warmer climates. In order to live in harmony with the environment, one should eat foods grown in the environment—at least as much as possible. Denny said that one should keep the house cool, so that one can respond naturally and adapt to the cooler temperatures of winter. In this way, we become more yang, and so better able to adjust to the elements and the season.

"Well, I think we've taken this to the ridiculous extreme," I said. "Why don't we go all the way and pitch a tent out back?"

Denny smiled and advised me to wear a heavier sweater. Many nights I didn't take off my coat during dinner.

By mid-November, I needed to escape from the many pressures in my life—my cancer, my colleagues, and macrobiotics. I decided to spend Thanksgiving in Puerto Rico; a vacation would be medicinal, I thought. I would be gone a week and decided to have my apartment painted while I was away.

The macrobiotic community was planning a big Thanksgiving feast, and at dinner the week before Denny invited me to come. I told him I was going to Puerto Rico for the holiday. He asked me to reconsider. "How will you be able to eat?" he asked me.

"I'll find a natural foods restaurant. Surely, there's brown rice on the island, Denny," I assured him.

On the Friday before Thanksgiving, I flew to Puerto Rico and got a room at the Sheraton Hotel. Soon, I found a natural foods restaurant that served fried brown rice and vegetables. Judy Waxman would have fainted, to be sure, had she seen the quality of the food, but I told myself that I was only staying a short time and would survive it. For a couple of days I ate at this restaurant while I lounged on the beach and did a little sightseeing. My spirits soared. It was good to be away from it all and wonderful to be in the warm sun. I forgot about my illness, my colleagues, macrobiotics, and cold houses. A warm beach and the sound of the ocean in the back of one's mind can make one forget even death.

By Sunday evening I had gotten tired of the natural foods place and decided to have dinner in the hotel restaurant. I took a cold shower, dressed, and went down to the restaurant ready to indulge myself. I ordered the bouillabaisse, a fish stew. The meal was well prepared and tasted delicious. For about an hour and a half I sat there enjoying the meal and later a cool Perrier water. I relished the thought of returning to my old sensual and extravagant diet. I wallowed in the freedom of being able to go out to a restaurant and eat something forbidden.

The next morning I got out of bed and vomited profusely. I was feverish and achy. I spent all Monday hoping the nausea and diarrhea would pass. By Tuesday morning I decided to return to Philadelphia. All I wanted was to get into my own bed. I got an early flight out of Puerto Rico bound for home.

When I arrived at my apartment, the painter was still hard at work. My bedroom was only half finished, and the smell of paint fumes was everywhere. I could hardly breathe without my stomach doing somersaults.

The painter said he would be finished by Wednesday, which had been the agreed-upon deadline. I went to the nearest Holiday Inn and slept till late the next morning. After I got back to my apartment the following day I made myself a bowl of miso soup, with vegetables and wakame seaweed. For the first time since I started the macrobiotic diet, I actually enjoyed miso soup. Later I began to feel better and made myself some oatmeal and lentil beans. I debated whether I should call Denny and tell him I was back in town. I couldn't. I was too embarrassed to admit that I was back in Philadelphia, sick.

At about three Thursday afternoon, Thanksgiving, I went to the Japan House, a local restaurant that serves boiled and fried brown rice, vegetables, and occasionally miso soup. The Japan House is a small, basement restaurant with perhaps fifteen tables stationed along the walls and in the center of its dining room. Japanese lanterns hang from the ceiling and cast a pale glow. When I arrived, there was not a soul in the restaurant except me, the cook, and one waitress. No one had been in all day, I was told. And no one entered while I was there. I ordered rice and vegetables and ate with my chopsticks. As I ate I stared at my meal, while the waitress had nothing to do but stare at me.

The next day I went back to eating my meals with the Waxmans and I put the Japan House and Puerto Rico behind me. However, during the first few weeks in December I began to lose weight rapidly. I had lost a few pounds in November, but by December the weight loss became dramatic. Weight loss in cancer patients is normally associated with advancement of cancer, and I started to worry. Soon, I dropped from 165 pounds to 135. By the middle of December I thought the cancer was running wild inside me. Oddly enough, I felt well otherwise. This did not seem to make sense in light of the weight reduction, which in cancer patients is associated with muscle-wasting, fatigue, and sometimes depression.

I went to Sheldon Lisker and had an examination and some blood tests performed, all of which showed that there was no progression of the cancer. Sheldon told me not to worry about the weight, but that we should continue to follow my condition closely.

"Sheldon, I've been following a vegetarian diet," I said. "It's called macrobiotics — mostly grains, some cooked vegetables, beans, and seaweed. These people seem to think that it might be beneficial in the treatment of cancer."

"Why don't you tell me about it, Tony," Sheldon said.

I gave Sheldon a very cursory explanation of macrobiotics. He questioned me closely on the nutritional value of the diet and finally said that he saw no harm in the regimen as long as I made sure I was getting adequate nutrients and calories and it did not interfere with the treatment I was receiving. He said that he saw no basis for any claims that macrobiotics might be of benefit to cancer patients, but there was no harm in followng the diet. Overall, he was very supportive, and told me to keep him informed of how I was eating. We then parted.

After I had seen Sheldon, Denny examined me closely and also assured me that all was well.

"But, Denny, I'm losing all this weight. Pretty soon I'll be able to hide behind my stethoscope."

He agreed that normally weight loss is a bad sign. But in my case it was a reflection of my body coming back into balance. I was shedding a lot of excess in my body, especially that put on as a result of the estrogens, Denny said.

I was feeling well at Christmas time and decided to risk another trip. My parents had usually gone to New Smyrna Beach, Florida, at Christmas. I wanted my mother to stay in the habit of making the annual trip. It would do her good to get away from Long Beach Island and spend time in the sun, I decided. I would be staying at her apartment, so I would not have to rely on restaurants for food. My mother, who by now had long known about the macrobiotic diet, assured me that she would cook macrobiotic meals while we were in Florida together. My only concern was whether the Auto-train, which we had planned to ride to Florida, would serve fish in its dining car. We were told when we made reservations that they would have fish.

On December 26, my mother and I drove to Washington, D.C., and got on the Autotrain. That night we went to the dining car and ordered, only to be told that they had just run out of fish. I ordered chicken instead. Within two days, I got a repeat performance of Puerto Rico: vomiting, diarrhea, aches and pains, and continual nausea. Worst of all, the pain in my back returned.

For the next few days in Florida, I ate very simply and most of the symptoms disappeared. The pain in my back — though considerably less severe than it had been — remained, however. I decided to stay in Florida until after New Year's.

On New Year's Eve, I went out on the town. I drove to a strip of bars in Daytona Beach and hung out for a few hours talking with some people I had met. I bought a beer and took perhaps three sips of it while I made conversation. Later, on impulse I drove my car to the beach and got stuck in some sand. I had another beer in my hand as I walked down by the ocean. I sat in the sand by the water and looked out into the night. The sky was overcast, but the clouds were broken so that at intervals the moon showed through. The ocean was black as death. All I could see were the breaking waves some fifty feet out. Beyond that, nothing.

"Happy New Year," I called out to the void. "It's been one hell of a year."

I took a swallow of beer and said to myself, "If this beer makes the cancer come back, then to hell with it. It's New Year's."

Chapter 8

WHEN I RETURNED to Philadelphia, I knew I could not go on eating exclusively with the Waxmans. I had grown used to many of the nuances and idiosyncrasies of the macrobiotic practice. I no longer felt awkward eating with chopsticks, for example, and the food was becoming palatable to me, some of it even enjoyable. But I did not feel comfortable with my dependence upon the Waxman family. I was very grateful for all that they were doing for me, but I needed a greater sense of freedom.

Denny was very understanding of my feelings and recommended several families (among the several hundred macrobiotic people in the greater Philadelphia area) with whom I could eat and not worry about the quality of the cooking. Soon, I began to widen my circle of macrobiotic friends.

Eating with other people in the community opened my eyes to the diversity with which macrobiotics could be practiced. I discovered that people interpreted the form of macrobiotics quite differently from one another. Of those with whom I ate, no one veered from the substance of macrobiotics—that is, they maintained the standard diet and applied the philosophy of yin and yang—but most people determined for themselves how they would incorporate the discipline into their lives. Not everyone sat on the floor, for example, nor did everyone eat with chopsticks. Many people stayed with their traditional religious roots, whether they were Christian or Jewish, while others took up an Eastern philosophy or created their own personal form of spiritual expression.

What they all seemed to share was a basic respect and gratitude for the food. This sprang from a sense that food had a spiritual origin; that is, it was very much a gift from God and one acknowledged this by giving thanks. I also recognized the deep and abiding faith that these people maintained in the healing power of food. Everywhere I went I was reassured that if I continued to eat well I could reverse my cancer.

Seeing this diversity within the community did much for my willingness to stick with macrobiotics. It didn't have to be as foreign to me as it initially seemed. As the leader of the community, Denny tended to maintain a form and standards that appeared to me more doctrinaire than those of some of the other practitioners.

Nevertheless, despite this diversity in the style, I was able to maintain a strict macrobiotic diet. Apart from my two indiscretions—the trip to Puerto Rico and the chicken at Christmas time—I didn't veer from the diet prescribed by Michio Kushi and Denny Waxman: 50 percent whole grains; 25 to 30 percent vegetables; 15 percent beans and sea vegetables, and the rest condiments and soups. As I mentioned earlier my only variation from the standard diet came in volume. I was able to maintain the diet through will power and my own inherent discipline. I also had the added incentive of fearing that if I went off the diet I would soon be dead.

Once I reversed my condition, Denny assured me that I could widen my diet without harmful effects. This wider diet, which most macrobiotic people were on, included fish and various macrobiotic desserts, including natural sweeteners such as fruit, barley malt, and rice syrup.

It wasn't long before I recovered from my trip to Florida. The back pain had persisted, however, and I was concerned that the cancer had begun to spread along my spinal column where I already had a lesion. I went back to Denny for his opinion; I planned to see Sheldon Lisker soon, as well.

Denny met me in his study and gave me the same thorough examination that by now I had grown accustomed to. When he had finished he said that everything was fine. I was progressing rapidly.

"Why do I still have the back pain, then?" I asked. "Couldn't this indicate that the cancer is awakening after a period of dormancy?"

"Not in your case. The pain you are suffering from now is from blockage in the bladder meridian. I don't believe it's bone pain."

"What is the bladder meridian? Are you talking about acupuncture meridians?"

At this point Denny launched off into another one of his lengthy explanations that seemed to contradict everything in Western medicine and left me more dumfounded and skeptical than ever.

He proceeded to tell me that each of us has twelve meridians, or channels of energy, that flow vertically throughout the body. The macrobiotic theory is that each meridian feeds energy to various organs. The meridians run just below the surface of the skin and go to great depths within the body, like twelve deep rivers of energy. The energy that passes along each meridian originates from heaven and earth. From heaven there is solar and stellar electromagnetic energy, which radiates downward upon the earth. The earth's energy radiates upward and is caused by the earth's rotation, which also generates electromagnetic energy. The energy from heaven showers down upon us and is taken in mostly through the top of our heads. Earth's energy is taken in through the bottom of the feet and the genitals.

There are seven major areas between the head and the feet where these two charges meet. These seven zones are called chakras, and they correspond to major organs and glands where the forces of heaven and earth collide with one another, thus stimulating certain areas of our bodies with additional energy. These seven chakras are: a point at the top of the head where the hair spirals; the mid-brain; the throat; the heart; the stomach; a place called hara that Denny called the seat of the will, located in the center of the intestines below the navel; and the sex organs.

According to macrobiotic theory, this energy from heaven and earth, sometimes called ki in the East, is what gives us life. Waxman went on to say that when a meridian is blocked or there is stagnation along its path, it is like having a big rock stuck in a river. Energy gets backed up and there is pain and soreness. That's the origin of your pain, he told me.

"How do you know? How do you know this is bladder meridian pain and not bone pain?" I asked, assuming in spite of myself that there might be some logic to his theories.

"Because your cancer is in remission," he said confidently.

"And how do you know that?"

By looking at my meridians, Denny said, he could see various discolorations, moles, pimples, or other signs that show problems with the corresponding organs. My meridians were clearing, he said. Also, there are several points on the face that correspond to organs within the body, and these too indicated that my cancer was receding. He said that if I applied a ginger compress to my back over the area of the pain, it would go away. The ginger compress would unblock a lot of stagnation.*

As a medical doctor, I found all of this to be preposterous and would have dropped the whole business then and there except that, for whatever reasons, I knew the diet seemed to have greatly improved my health.

I was faced with an enormous conflict. Was macrobiotics pure charlatanism, an utter fake—something I could not help but believe at times—or was it a view of healing and reality with which the West had not yet come to grips? I seemed to be constantly oppressed by this question. The fact that I am a doctor seemed to complicate matters further for me. As a patient, all I had to worry about was how I felt; but as a doctor, I was continually wrestling with the possibility that I might have discovered something that could be of benefit to mankind. Out of this latter role came the necessity that I prove as far as I could—through my own experience—that macrobiotics was right about health and disease.

Denny's comment that my cancer was in remission was yet another macrobiotic claim that I was compelled to test. I had been scheduled to have a full series of blood and liver-function tests done at Methodist shortly after our conversation, and if my cancer was indeed regressing, the tests would indicate such a change.

On January 22, I had the tests performed. The following day the results were delivered to Sheldon Lisker, who went over them with me. Eight months before, on May 31, 1978, my blood and liver-function studies indicated the presence of cancer. The alkaline phosphatase level in my blood was 69; normal is anywhere between 9 and 35. My SGOT and SGPT, both liver-function tests and both key indicators

*I would later learn that the ginger compress could not be used indiscriminately with cancer, because the compress sometimes caused the cancer to spread. Waxman felt, however, that I had progressed far enough to begin using the ginger compress.

for cancer, were 100 and 273, respectively. The normal range for both tests is between 13 and 40. All of these tests indicated the presence of a well-differentiated cancer.

On January 23, however, there were some notable changes. My alkaline phosphatase level had dropped to 36; the SGOT had dropped to 21; and my SGPT had gone down to 27. My condition had improved dramatically!

Sheldon attributed the improvement to the orchiectomy and the estrogen treatment. He said that these were good signs and admitted that they were somewhat out of the ordinary. Sheldon was cautious in his interpretation of the test results, since this did not mean that the cancer was eliminated, or even in the process of remission. It simply meant that the disease might have been temporarily arrested. We would have to wait and see what happened next.

It was impossible to draw any firm conclusions on the basis of these tests. They were just laboratory studies, and the only way to know the status of my cancer for sure was to take a bone scan, but there was no medical reason at this point to do such a test. Moreover, cancer patients often experience a period of apparent improvement and then take a turn for the worse. My father followed this pattern; for a few weeks after his initial surgery, he seemed to be well. Then suddenly his condition worsened and the outcome rarely seemed in doubt.

Nevertheless, I was encouraged by the test results. They were one more piece of evidence that seemed to support other small clues that suggested my condition was improving. I had read the studies on this type of carcinoma and my pattern seemed unique. At first I had enormous back pain, which is normal, and I gained a considerable amount of weight from the estrogens, also normal. However, within weeks after beginning macrobiotics, my back pain vanished.

This occurred more than a month after I had been taking estrogens without a reduction in pain. The estrogens may have had a delayed reaction and in fact been responsible for the pain relief. The fact that I had been practicing macrobiotics at that point may have only been coincidental to the relief of the pain, but somehow I doubted that was the case. Shortly after the pain subsided, the weight from the estrogens began to leave me. This had seemed a clear indication that the cancer was advancing and my period of improvement was at an end. However, exactly the opposite seemed to occur. My weight stabilized and I gained back ten pounds. Moreover, I continued to feel strong and generally positive. This is not characteristic of an advancing carcinoma.

When Sheldon and I finished going over the tests, I very cautiously asked him if he thought the diet I had been on was in any way responsible for my improvement.

"No, Tony. There's no scientific evidence that I'm aware of which suggests diet plays any role in the treatment of cancer. At least not the kind of role you're talking about."

"Well, there may not be any evidence to support the hypothesis, Sheldon, but I'm beginning to believe that this diet is helping me," I said. "I don't know how it's doing it, but I feel much better, beyond what you might attribute to the recovery from surgery."

"Well, certainly your positive attitude could be of benefit in your treatment, but I can't say that your attitude has anything to do with the diet," Sheldon said.

I then explained the macrobiotic view that the mind and body are one. That is, as I ate better and felt physically stronger and healthier, my attitude toward my circumstances became more positive. My positive attitude, coupled with a healthier diet, helped me to better fight the cancer. In other words, macrobiotics was offering the age-old axiom that a healthy body makes a healthy mind, and vice versa. It was simply saying that you could begin this cycle with a good diet.

Sheldon did not try to close the door on my theories, nor on my incipient enthusiasm for macrobiotics. He simply said again that he believed my progress was due to the orchiectomy and the estrogens.

We then discussed my back pain, which he said was a recurrence of the bone pain. Sheldon suggested I resume the Percodan, which I did on a periodic, though less frequent, basis.

I left Sheldon's office that day still deeply skeptical of macrobiotics, but nevertheless holding on to some fragile hope that in some way I was being miraculously healed.

I didn't realize then how fragile that hope really was.

One night early in February I awoke at about 2 A.M. I got up and went into the bathroom and began urinating profusely. This happened a couple of times in the same night. The next morning I got up and once again had an extended urination. Otherwise I felt fine. I went to the office, but by nine-thirty I had developed a lower back pain. By ten it was excruciating and by eleven I had a massive kidney attack. X-rays revealed that I was passing a kidney stone, and I was given an injection of morphine to reduce the pain. Initially, I believed I would need surgery to remove the stone, but in an hour the stone passed.

I went back to my office and telephoned Denny Waxman and called him every name in the book. I had never had a kidney stone in my life and I was sure that the macrobiotic diet had caused it. I was finally seeing the negative effects of the diet, I believed. I yelled at Denny for several minutes. When I finished, he said, "Tony, can I come down to your office to talk to you?" Still angry, I agreed to see him, thinking that we would put an end to our relationship then.

When he entered my office, he very calmly stated that the

kidney stone was an excellent sign. "The stone is a form of discharge, Tony. It's really a sign of deep healing."

He went on to say that the kidneys were cleansing the blood of toxins that were being discharged from my body. Also the toxins that had been accumulating in the kidneys over the years were being discharged. In this instance, it came out in the form of a stone.

I had calmed down considerably by then and I wanted to believe him. On some emotional level what he was saying made sense. He had told me before I began the diet that there would be various forms of discharge; the symptoms of the flu, which I had in September, were only the first round and there would be others later on.

"You're sure about this?" I asked.

"Yes. Don't worry. See how you feel over the next few weeks."

Feeling a bit sheepish about my emotional outburst, I agreed to wait before I gave up on the diet. Still, I was plunged into another deep bout of skepticism. Despite the definite signs of progress I had made, I was always being followed by the shadow of doubt, which engulfed me every time a situation arose that did not correspond with my own medical understanding. As far as I was concerned, the world of macrobiotics did not necessarily exist under the same physical laws as those I took as second nature. My logic and my knowledge were being turned upside down, and the only reason I persisted in letting this happen was the small hope that it might save my life. Once again I decided to reserve judgment.

Of course, part of my problem with macrobiotics—aside from my major intellectual differences with it—was my feeling that I was practicing it all alone. There was no one within my peer group, especially no physician, to whom I could go for reassurance. Although I would later learn that there are a number of physicians around the country practicing this way of life, I did not know of any then. As a result, I felt utterly alone in my efforts to bridge the gap between my Western medical training and this Eastern, philosophically based system. Feeling isolated only served to reinforce my skepticism. This diet and philosophy is only fit for the kooks, I often thought. The kooks and this desperate doctor dying of cancer.

One night at an East West Foundation lecture, I met Bob and Sylvia Roberman. The Robermans were my own age. Bob was a successful stockbroker and Sylvia a registered nurse. Both had lived in Philadelphia most of their lives. A couple of weeks after we met, I accepted their invitation to dinner.

The Robermans were a handsome couple. Sylvia was about five feet six inches tall, with short, dark brown hair and a heart-shaped face. Her eyes were large and brown and her nose and mouth small. Sylvia impressed me the moment I met her as having the energy of someone twenty years her junior. She was assertive and prone to speak her mind.

Bob had a quiet and mannered confidence. He was a handsome man, with a slender, athletic build. He was an inch shorter than his wife.

They lived in a lovely apartment in the suburbs of Philadelphia. They had obviously done well in life. I had grown curious about what brought people to macrobiotics, particularly those who were in my own age group and with my social background.

Sylvia served a simple meal the night I joined them for dinner. She made pressure-cooked brown rice, lentil soup, greens with a tofu dressing, and steamed cauliflower and carrots. As we ate I asked them why they had come to macrobiotics.

Sylvia took the question first. For years she had been suffering from hemorrhagic bleeding at the time of her period and was in a deep depression. She was taking up to nineteen pills a day for both conditions, including lithium, triaville, Valium, ferasulfate, and vitamin pills. "I was a wreck," she said. "And meanwhile I was paying the best psychiatrist in Philadelphia a fortune to listen to me once a week and I wasn't getting any better. I was miserable."

At that time, her daughter was quietly practicing macrobiotics in their kitchen. The daughter occasionally suggested her mother take up this diet and see if it wouldn't help. Sylvia decided to try it. "Why not?" she said. "I had tried everything else." That was the fall of 1976.

Sylvia claimed that within two months she cleaned out her medicine cabinet. She said she felt wonderful. Meanwhile, the hemorrhagic bleeding gradually disappeared. "A few months after I started macrobiotics I stopped having the extreme depression, and I haven't been depressed at all in I don't know how long," she said. "I haven't taken a pill in two years."

"And you've come along for the ride, right?" I said to Bob.

"No, no," he said, smiling. "No, I had my problems, too. I was impotent."

He went to a number of physicians and psychiatrists, but nothing seemed to work. He began macrobiotics with his wife. It took him six months before he began to improve; within a year he claimed the condition was virtually eliminated.

"I would not have believed it, really," he said. They told him that the meridians in the lower part of his body were clogged with fat. This resulted in a loss of vitality, not only with the sex organs, but with the functions of all his lower organs. He said he had had trouble urinating and with bowel elimination. "After we had been practicing macrobiotics for a few months, all of this was improved," he said.

"This is not a panacea," said Bob. "We're not claiming that a good diet will undo every social ill, or make anyone a perfect person—even perfectly healthy, if there is such a state. But we feel this is the only sane way to eat, especially at our ages."

"Food is the basis," said Sylvia. "Macrobiotics will give you improved health. It's up to you to do something with it. The food is not going to change your life for you."

No matter where I went for dinner, people had similar anecdotes to report. Although I was suspicious of all of them, I was encouraged by their accounts. They meant nothing scientifically; they were individual reports that could not be substantiated or proved in any way. What they were for me was hope. These people claimed to have surmounted difficult circumstances through a positive attitude and the use of macrobiotics. I was hoping that I could do the same.

By March I was ready to attempt another trip. This time I planned it around the macrobiotic community in Miami, Florida. Mona Schwartz, the woman I had met at my first cooking class with Judy Waxman, had invited me there and I took her up on the invitation. In the middle of the month, I flew to Miami and stayed at the Coconut Grove, which is near the East West Center. I ate my meals with Mona and at the Oak Feed, a local macrobiotic restaurant.

The trip was wonderful. Between Mona's hospitality and the Oak Feed restaurant, I had no trouble eating good-quality macrobiotic food. I left Florida realizing that if I planned it right, I could travel throughout the country and even to Europe, where Michio had said there were hundreds of East West Centers. I love to travel, and my sense of freedom was being restored. The feeling that I was being trapped by macrobiotics was fading.

In the middle of April, I had another series of blood and liver-function tests done: there was no laboratory evidence of cancer in my body. At this point, I felt we really had something and I said as much to Sheldon.

"Sheldon, I'm convinced that this macrobiotic diet has

something to do with my progress. Half the ideas sound crazy, but some of them may be right." I then told Sheldon a little bit about the macrobiotic concepts of balance, discharge and accumulation, and the healing power of food. I said that the macrobiotic people believe that health depends on one's entire system being in a state of balance. I explained that this balance depended upon the kinds of foods that were taken into the body. The macrobiotic view holds that the body can handle a certain limited amount of toxins being taken in through the food. So long as these toxins remain below certain levels, the body can discharge them through the normal means of elimination. When this limit is exceeded, however, the body begins to accumulate the toxins in various places, mostly in the arteries and around the heart, as well as within certain organs. This accumulation ultimately results in various kinds of illnesses, including cardiovascular disease and cancer, which represent an extreme imbalance within the body, depending upon the kinds of foods that predominated in the diet. The macrobiotic people maintain that this process of degeneration and accumulation can be reversed through a diet that is free of these toxic elements; by eliminating insulting constituents from the diet, the process of accumulation can not only be stopped, but actually reversed. The body naturally discharges the toxins from the system, and thus frees itself from the cause of disease. The body returns to a state of balance, and health.

As I spoke, Sheldon looked at me with genuine curiosity and respect. He did not seem uninterested or threatened. He simply sat there with that same open, alert expression that I had come to know so well. Still, I had not forgotten how I reacted to these ideas when I first heard Denny discuss them.

"I realize this sounds crazy, Sheldon," I said. "But I'm noticing a lot of changes taking place in my own body and these tests seem to confirm that something positive is happening to me. All of this sounds even crazier if we talk about yin and yang and ki flow and all the rest that makes up the macrobiotic view," I continued. "But what I'm beginning to feel is that these macrobiotic people understand healing, and life in general, in philosophical and metaphorical terms, while we doctors and scientists see things in scientific and analytical frameworks. Neither one may be wrong; they're simply different ways of looking at the same condition. The macrobiotic view may well complement the scientific approach, and vice versa."

"Well, Tony, this is all very interesting," Sheldon said. "And I'm open to hearing more about macrobiotics, but as your doctor I must say again that there is no scientific or medical basis for what you are saying, and so I can't support macrobiotics as having any therapeutic value. On the other hand, you seem to be doing very well; I think this improvement is due to the orchiectomy and the estrogens, but the diet does not seem to be hurting you in any way. If anything, it seems to have given you a reason for hope and contributed to your positive attitude. You seem to have some faith in it, so I encourage you to continue what you're doing. Let's just continue to watch it."

Sheldon recommended that I have laboratory tests done every three months. I was glad to have the frank talk with him about my unconventional regimen and I left his office feeling very positive and extremely hopeful. On top of the laboratory results, I noticed that I seemed to be looking younger of late. The color of my face seemed brighter, and my skin tighter. The heavy jowls that I had had, as well as the bags beneath my eyes, were disappearing. I didn't look like a man dying of cancer. Furthermore, I felt a deep sense of well-being.

I was filled with hope and optimism. Clearly, there seemed some medical support for the macrobiotic claim that I was getting better. Maybe, just maybe, they were right. Perhaps there was something to the use of diet as a treatment for cancer.

As April turned into May, spring stretched out of its somnolence and, in a way, so did I. Something deep inside me told me that I had turned the corner, that I was on my way to recovery. There was a release of joy from within, a feeling that all my vital energies were no longer being dedicated solely to the battle against this disease. I had broken through. I felt like a bird on the wing.

Chapter 9

ON THE SECOND Saturday in June, I drove to the East West Foundation's Mid-Atlantic Summer Camp in Phoenixville, Pennsylvania, about an hour northwest of Philadelphia. The camp, which provided macrobiotic instruction in health and natural healing, was organized by Murray Snyder, director of the East West Foundation in Baltimore, and Denny Waxman. I arrived at the campgrounds in the pine-studded hills outside of Phoenixville just before noon. Murray met me and showed me around.

Like Denny Waxman, Murray had been a student of Michio Kushi's for about ten years. He is about six feet tall, with black hair, small brown eyes, and a ruddy, healthy-looking complexion. Murray has an enthusiastic, even inspiring, personality; with the way I was feeling, we couldn't have been more in harmony.

The campsite was in a valley surrounded by a forest that crept up the sides of some gradual hills. It was a peaceful and rustic setting, composed of three main buildings, where the classes were given, and several cabins where people slept. Many of those attending the camp pitched tents in the grassy field nearby.

About two hundred people were present for the week-long camp, Murray said. Most of them were from Pennsylvania, New York, Maryland, New Jersey, and Florida. Many were new to macrobiotics, but the majority were veterans of brown rice and miso soup.

The sky was clear the afternoon I arrived and there was a lot of enthusiasm loose in the air. I was excited to see Michio.

Soon Murray directed me to where Michio was giving a class at one of the buildings on the grounds. Michio and I agreed to meet later, and at about 3 P.M. I drove out to Phoenixville to meet him at his hotel. As I drove, I felt old doubts closing in on me. There I was, on my way to see a man who would look at me and tell me the status of my cancer. Part of me insisted that this was ridiculous. In fact, I was never able to reconcile my practice of macrobiotics with some aspects of my nature and my medical background. Some part of me insisted that the whole system — if indeed it could be called a system — seemed like sheer madness. Yet, I could not discount the fact that so long as I stayed on this crazy diet, the impossible — or at least the improbable — was happening to me. I didn't quite know how to deal with this conflict within me except to go on. Meanwhile, I kept waiting for the fairy godmother's golden coach to turn into a pumpkin.

For this reason, I never fully left the guidance of my medical colleagues. Paradoxically, they only gave me more faith in macrobiotics, since my medical tests tended to confirm some of the things the macrobiotic people were telling me in advance. I had already decided to meet with Sheldon Lisker within a couple of days for more blood tests and to discuss my progress.

But right now my whole mind was focused on my meeting with Michio Kushi. Macrobiotics had become my reason for hope; it was the thread from which my life hung, and though I often thought that it was no more reason for hope than was the remote chance of a miracle, I was now beginning to believe that a miracle was on its way.

When I arrived at Michio's hotel room, Denny Waxman, Michael Rossoff, and Shizuko Yamamoto—a macrobiotic consultant from New York City—were waiting with him. Michio gave me a warm greeting, and I shook hands with Denny, Michael, and Shizuko. I hadn't seen Michael Rossoff since that day in October 1978 when I first met him and Michio at the Kushi house in Brookline. I had met Shizuko some months before in New York and had talked to her a couple of times since then. She is about forty years old and short, perhaps five feet two or three inches, a strongly built woman who, not surprisingly, is an expert in Shiatsu, or meridian, massage. She had even written a book on massage, entitled *Barefoot Massage.* Michio asked me if I had any objections if his three guests remained in the room while he examined me, and of course I didn't.

The others sat in chairs around a small, round table that was near the windows, while Michio pulled open the curtain and let in the afternoon sun. The room was typical in nearly every way: a double bed, carpeted floor, and some wooden chairs around a small table. The room was larger than many of those of other motels, however, and the walls were covered in a pleasant off-white paper.

Michio began to examine me. Everyone was a bit tense, it seemed to me, though I was clearly the most anxious. He peered into my eyes and asked me to look up, down, left, and right. He then examined my face closely and began probing the upper parts of my body.

He was dressed as he always is, in his dark blue, three-piece suit, white shirt, and silver and navy print tie. I searched his face for a clue to what he might be thinking but there was nothing there that might give away his thoughts. He could just as easily have been fitting me for a suit, for all his face revealed. A small fire started in the pit of my stomach.

I had been practicing macrobiotics for ten months by now. I had followed the regimen as closely as anyone could, I believed. Each night before I went to bed I considered my chances of surviving. I seemed to allow myself better odds with the passing of every month. Apart from the occasional back pain, which was not nearly as severe or as persistent as it had been, I had never felt so well in my life. I slept well at night and awoke refreshed and ready for the day. In the morning I did some yoga exercises that Denny had shown me. I felt strong throughout the day, without that midafternoon slump that I had grown so accustomed to. My mind was lucid and I seemed to be in better control of my emotions of late. I could lick this disease, I thought.

Michio asked me to roll up my sleeves and take off my shoes and socks. What exactly is he seeing? I asked myself. Was this stuff about meridians really true? Occasionally Michio would probe an area of my body with his thumb and issue a low growl from the back of his throat. He didn't say a word while he examined me. Everyone was silent. The tension started to build in my shoulders and I could feel that my breathing had gotten shorter.

It had been just twelve months before that I was told that I had a terminal illness. I believed then that I would be dead before my fiftieth birthday. What followed that diagnosis was a series of tragedies: three operations, the loss of my testicles, the death of my father, the slow dismantling of my mother, and the long and bitter wait for my own imminent death. And then I picked up two hitchhikers. Now today.

Soon Michio finished examining me and stood back. He looked at me in the way one does when one wants to remember someone's face.

"You don't have cancer anymore, Tony. You've beaten your disease," Michio said. With that he stood back and smiled.

Suddenly a wall of tension, desperation, pain, and disappointment collapsed; joy rushed through me like healing waters. Everyone in the room was patting me on the back and congratulating me. I had done the impossible! I had licked a disease that was unbeatable by every measure I had believed in.

"I knew it, I knew it," I said. I could feel the happiness bursting from my face. "I know I'm well, by God!"

The room was filled with a kind of giddy joy for a few more moments. When the energy died down some, Michio said, "You're not completely out of danger yet, Tony. You need time and continued good eating."

At first I was taken aback. He appeared to be contradicting himself. Then he explained that, in the macrobiotic view, cancer takes seven years to be purged from the body. During that time, every cell in the body is replaced, and the cancer is fully discharged. I was now out of immediate danger and on the surface all was well; however, I could easily have a relapse if I changed my lifestyle and diet. I must be careful of how I eat and live, Michio said, particularly over the next few years.

We then discussed the treatment I was undergoing, particularly the estrogens. I told him I was feeling very well, under the circumstances, and appeared to be getting stronger week by week. Michio said that I could get well with or without the estrogens, although in my own case the estrogens might slow my recovery somewhat because they created an imbalance in the body that would take time to rectify. According to macrobiotic theory, estrogens — being the female hormone — are more yin than other hormones, and thus upset the body's attempt to return to a balanced condition. Michio said that the balance could be restored if I remained on the estrogens, but it would take far longer. We discussed my going off them, and it was left up to me to make the decision.

I asked him when he believed I could successfully undergo a bone scan. I desperately wanted to have one as soon as possible to know for sure if I had indeed beaten the cancer.

"The test is dangerous, Tony," Michio said. "You know that radioactive dye is not on the macrobiotic diet."

"I've got to know for sure, and the test is the only way to do that," I said. "When do you think I could safely have the test done and come out of it with a clean bill of health?"

Michio was naturally a little hurt that my faith seemed so shallow. But I felt the need to document my recovery medically. The medical profession would not accept Michio's word that I was well, and I was always conscious of what my recovery would mean to others if I had strong evidence that diet could be effective in the treatment of cancer. My recovery would mean little beyond what it meant to me personally without all the medical documentation I could provide.

Michio asked me to wait till November or December before having a bone scan. Disappointed and feeling a vague sense of unease, I turned to another subject. "When can I widen my diet?" I asked.

"In six months," was Michio's answer. "At that time add a little fruit a couple of times a week. A little later you can take a small portion of fish once a week, but let's wait for a while on the fish."

Michio then asked me if it would be all right if he made an announcement at the gathering that night concerning my recovery, adding that it would encourage many people to get well. I allowed this, so long as he said there was no medical evidence as yet that I had reversed my disease.

Michio then gave me a warm smile and said, "I predict today, Tony, that you will be responsible for saving a million lives."

That statement—shocking as it sounded to me—set off another round of congratulations and reignited the joy in the room. Once again I was aware of my enormous relief and happiness. For a few more minutes we all sat in the room and talked and I expressed my deepest gratitude to all of them, particularly to Denny and Michio, for the help they gave me. How does one adequately express his thanks to those who reached out and pulled him from the nether world of death? All I could say was thank you.

For the next few days I considered going off the estrogens. I had been practicing macrobiotics all this time, and I had apparently made great progress. Yet I never knew for sure whether that progress could be attributed to the diet or to the estrogens and the orchiectomy. Was I enduring this way of life for nothing, or was there really something to macrobiotics? Over the past several months, I had slowly come to suspect that my improvement had more to do with the macrobiotic approach than with the estrogens. By then I had learned enough about Oriental diagnosis to notice specific changes in my face, hands, and overall health. I was changing, there was no doubt of that. I was taking on a more youthful, vital appearance, which was accompanied by a general sense of well-being. I looked and felt better, and it was happening according to a pattern the macrobiotic people almost took for granted. Still, this is hardly proof of a useful cancer therapy.

Had I not been a doctor, my ambivalence toward macrobiotics and the estrogens might never have mattered; after all, I was getting better. But it did matter to me — it mattered a great deal. Despite the fact that I was now a patient, a part of me never stopped thinking like a doctor. I often wondered if the diet would have helped my father. I also wanted to test the diet and philosophy — insofar as was possible — because of the deeper implications it had on my own values as a human being. Were my previous diet and living habits the causes of my cancer? Short of the cancer itself, nothing in my life had ever turned so many of my values completely upside down in the way that macrobiotics had. I needed to know if this crazy system had any substance to it.

Of course, there was still the possibility that the orchiectomy could have been responsible for my improved health, but I strongly doubted this was the case. The disease was clearly regressing, I was quickly getting stronger, I had more energy than I had had in twenty years, and my pattern seemed inconsistent with the vast majority of cases of prostatic cancer, stage IV (D), which had been treated with orchiectomy and estrogens.

I decided the safest test I could perform on myself was to go off the estrogens. Following my decision, I went to Sheldon Lisker's office and discussed it with him. He was adamantly opposed to it.

"Tony, it is medically unadvisable for you to stop the estrogens now. You're doing well, and I'm very happy you're improving. But if you go off the estrogens, it's highly likely that your cancer will reemerge. This is a safe and effective treatment and one that might prolong your life. I feel very strongly that you should not be changing the therapy now."

"Sheldon, I think it's the diet that's responsible for my improved health. I've got to know for sure whether it's the diet or the estrogens."

At this point, I told Sheldon that I had seen Michio Kushi a few days before and that he had told me that I was doing well.

"Kushi thinks my cancer is almost gone," I said cautiously.

"Well, Tony, I'm glad to hear that your macrobiotic friends feel you're improving, but I cannot be a party to your going off the estrogen therapy," Sheldon said. The idea that I might be improving because of the macrobiotic diet was preposterous to Sheldon. He then reiterated that there was no medical evidence to suggest that diet could be an effective therapy for cancer. "I think you're playing with your life, Tony. I'm very opposed to your changing the treatment now."

I explained to Sheldon that I wanted to do it on a trial basis. "Let's see what happens. I'll keep a close watch on it and if anything happens I'll resume the estrogens."

He was clearly upset with me. Sheldon is one of those persons who never seem to be ruffled by anything, so that any small change in demeanor is impressive. He had now become firm and authoritative.

"I'm concerned that if the cancer flares up again we won't be able to slow its progress, even if you go back on the estrogens," Sheldon said. "You and I both realize there are no guarantees with this kind of thing; we may not be able to arrest it once the disease gets going again."

"Sheldon, I want to go off the estrogens for a month or two to see what happens. I want to see how I feel and whether there are any appreciable changes in my condition." I explained to him that I had radically changed my eating habits and lifestyle for macrobiotics and I had to know if there was any substance to it. I already had strong suspicions. As a doctor who might be in a position someday to be an advocate for a nutritional approach to disease and prevention, I felt I had to prove the efficacy of the diet as far as I could.

Sheldon paused a few moments and studied my face.

"Well, Tony, you are a physician and you know what you are doing. I'll go along with you. We'll just have to watch your condition very closely."

"Thanks, Sheldon," I said.

I discontinued my daily dosages of estrogen pills during the third week in June. I had resolved to wait until my next set of blood tests to see if there was any significant change in my condition. If it worsened, I would know that the estrogens were at least partly responsible for my improved health, and that the diet was not the sole cause of my apparent improvement. At that point I would resume the estrogens.

Throughout the summer I continued to feel strong and positive about my health. By the middle of August, my laboratory tests showed no appreciable change. My SGOT, SGPT, and LDH, all liver-function tests, rose a few points, to 28, 43, and 0.7 respectively. These were not indicative of the presence of cancer. I felt confident that my system was just reacting to the absence of the estrogens and that even the liver-function tests would eventually right themselves, though they were hardly abnormal where they were.

There was one side effect, however; I had hot flashes periodically as a result of the lack of testosterone or estrogen in my body, a condition one might say is analogous to male menopause. The hot flashes and sweating were minor and infrequent, however.

In the meantime, the East West Foundation held its annual Amherst Program at Amherst College in central Massachusetts during the last week in August. The Amherst Program was the foundation's premier conference. Over the years that it had been held, many noted physicians and scientists—though obviously skeptical—had attended to listen to the macrobiotic approach to cancer and other degenerative illnesses. In 1979, I was a guest of Michio Kushi's and at that year's program I met Jean Kohler.

Kohler was a Ph.D. and had been a professor of music at Ball State University in Muncie, Indiana, for some thirty years. He was an elfish, happy man, who had a midwesterner's dry wit and frank expression. He was sixty-one when I met him. Six years earlier, Kohler had been diagnosed as having cancer of the pancreas. In 1973, physicians at Indiana University Medical Center performed exploratory surgery on him and discovered a large tumor on his pancreas. The tumor was the size of a fist and had metastasized and spread to his duodenum. Pancreatic cancer is a death sentence. It is one of the most intractable cancers known today, and Kohler and his wife Mary Alice were told by his doctors that he had no hope of surviving. Nevertheless, his physicians encouraged him to take chemotherapy, and he took one treatment. Then a friend told him about macrobiotics. Shortly thereafter, Kohler had a consultation with Michio Kushi and began the macrobiotic diet. Within a year, his laboratory tests showed no sign of cancer and he claimed to be feeling fine. Over the next seven years, he made a crusade of telling people that he had cured cancer through a positive attitude and the macrobiotic diet. He wrote a book entitled *Healing Miracles Through Macrobiotics,* and lectured to audiences across the country.

When I met him, Kohler was the personification of positive thinking. I was greatly impressed and encouraged by him, and particularly by the fact that he was still alive to talk about such a devastating illness. For me, Kohler was yet another sign of hope.

Michio and I had a chance to spend some time together at Amherst and I told him that I was considering having the bone scan done in September. "No, don't have it done in September, Tony," Michio said. "There will be some small sign of the disease left. Why don't you wait till December. Then all will be fine."

But I was concerned with the need to get traditional medical corroboration for my apparent improvement and I couldn't wait till December. When I returned to Philadelphia, I immediately scheduled a bone scan for September 27 at Methodist Hospital.

The month of September passed quickly. I was moving around the hospital at full tilt, full of energy and charged with optimism. If this is what macrobiotic people call ki, then I was imbued with it. The change did not go unnoticed. People around the hospital began to come to me in private and ask me what I was doing that made me so energetic.

They had heard that I was on some weird diet; what was this macrobiotic regimen all about? I told them that I was experimenting with macrobiotics as a complement to the medical treatment I was receiving for cancer. I couldn't say for sure, but I believed that the diet was responsible for my increased vitality. I also explained a little about macrobiotics. My explanation drew a variety of responses, from mild interest to outright dismissal and dismay. Meanwhile, I kept my eye on the calendar.

A few days before I was scheduled to have the bone scan performed, I flew to Boston to have another consultation with Michio Kushi. I wanted to know how Michio thought the bone scan would go. We met at his house and Michio gave me a quick examination there. He then told me I was well.

"How do you think the bone scan will react, Michio?" I asked.

Michio said that there were still some small traces of cancer inside me but I was in the process of discharging it. It would take time, but the cancer was very small. He said that the bone scan would either detect tiny traces of cancer, in which case I should not be worried, or it would find no trace of malignancy at all. More than likely, he said, the bone scan would show me to be completely healed.

On September 27, I got out of bed at my usual six-thirty wake-up time, showered, dressed, and drove to the office. I prayed like a man on his way to the gallows. When I arrived at the hospital, I went down to the x-ray department, where Dr. Anthony Renzi injected the radioactive dye into my veins. Then we waited the three hours for the dye to spread throughout my system.

Meantime, Dr. Renzi came into my office and told me what he expected to find from the bone scan. He had the records of my previous bone scan and laboratory studies with him.

He started out by saying that I had made enormous

progress. "You've arrested the disease, Tony," he said, adding that my x-rays would unquestionably show no progression of the lesions, and that was "a very good sign." However, Renzi admonished me not to be disappointed when we found the disease in the same basic pattern that it was in on May 31, 1978. "Bones take a long time to heal, Tony," said Renzi. "They're very deep and we can't expect much change over fifteen months. If there are a lot of other lesions, we'll have to be concerned." He repeated, however, that he did not expect to find that the cancer had progressed. Renzi got out of his chair and smiled. "See you in a couple of hours. I'll be praying for you, Tony," he said.

"Thanks," I said.

When the three hours were up, I went down the hall to radiology. I changed into a hospital gown and lay down on the table. Once again I became terribly nervous.

I looked over at the bone scan. Between the scanner's heavy metal arms was the drumlike Geiger counter that would detect how the dye reacted in my body. When the dye came into the presence of a tumor, it gathered together to form large radioactive masses. When the bone scan detected these aggregated areas of radioactivity, it would set off a rapid clicking sound, similar to that emitted by a Geiger counter when it discovers some radioactive element.

I could also see how the dye reacted by looking over at the oscilloscope in the computer, which would show the area of my body that was being examined by the scanner. Cancer would show up on the oscilloscope as black patches wherever a tumor was located. On the other hand, if there was no cancer in my body, the bone scan would release a slow, monotonous beat and the oscilloscope would show that the dye had spread homogenously throughout my body. There would be no black patches, no wild clicking, as there had been fifteen months before. These were the signs I was hoping for.

While Renzi and his assistant were busy readying the bone scan, I thought about the last time I lay on this table and underwent this test, that day fifteen months earlier when the bone scan discovered that my body was riddled with cancer—tumors in my skull, left sixth rib, right shoulder, sternum, and spine. The memory of that day would burn in my consciousness for the rest of my life.

I looked again at the bone scan. Some irrational fear of the machine came over me. It was coldly objective. There was nothing forgiving in that machine. Its world was black and white: either you have cancer or you don't. And I knew it would search like a wild bloodhound until it ferreted out a tumor in me.

Yet, I was hopeful. I remembered Michio's diagnosis.

Renzi turned on the machine and immediately it began clicking out a slow, monotonous beat, picking up traces of radioactive particles in the air. When he brought the drum down over my head the beat picked up, responding to the radioactive dye in my body. However, it remained steady and normal. I immediately looked over at the oscilloscope and saw the x-raylike outline of my head; there was no black patch as there had been before. There was no tumor in my skull! My heart swelled with hope. Renzi manipulated the sensitive end of the machine from my head to my shoulder; again, there was no change in the beat of the clicks, and again no black patch in the oscilloscope. My shoulder was healed! Renzi moved the drum over my entire body from my head to my feet. He made deliberate passes over the areas where the cancer had shown up before: the skull, right shoulder, sternum, rib cage, spine, and genitals. As Renzi directed the bone scan, my heart, my mind, my entire being was riveted on the cadence of the clicks. Every time he changed the placement of the drum, I shifted my head to see the oscilloscope.

All was normal. The wild, manic beat that I had listened

to before never emerged. Nowhere in my body did the machine find any cancer cells. My bones were healed. The cancer was gone.

Renzi was shocked. I got off the table and more x-rays were taken of my body. Still no sign of cancer. Renzi told me in amazement that he had never seen anything like this before. He didn't know what else to say or do but congratulate me. According to all the tests, I was perfectly healthy.

I was overcome with joy. I gave Tony Renzi a big bear hug. We clapped one another on the back and I cried out, "These macrobiotic people may sound crazy, Tony, but they've got something!"

"I don't know what you're doing, Tony," Renzi said to me. "But by God keep doing it."

Later that afternoon I took my x-ray results over to Sheldon Lisker's office, and he and I went over them together. He was also astounded. Like Renzi, he expected to find little change in the basic pattern of the disease. He was happily surprised.

"Tony, I'm very happy about this, though I want to caution you that we should continue to watch your progress," Sheldon said. "Still, from all the tests you're fine. I want to congratulate you."

Sheldon smiled and shook my hand. For a few minutes we talked about the previous fifteen months and how difficult a period it had been in my life.

"Sheldon, what do you think caused this change in my condition?" I asked.

"Frankly, Tony, I don't know. I can only assume that it was the therapy — the orchiectomy and the estrogens — that triggered your autoimmune system to fight off the cancer."

"Have you ever seen another case like mine?" I asked.

"No, I haven't," he said. "I'd say that your case is rare; I do understand that there are a few cases reported like this in the British literature. I think perhaps we might look at those cases to see what similarities there are."

"How does this affect the five-year survival rate?" I asked.

"Tony, we may as well throw those books out the window," Sheldon said. "When the bones are clean, where's the disease? We don't know what is going to happen to you from this point. That's why we've got to keep a watch over your condition."

Sheldon then said that he could not advise me to go off the macrobiotic diet or go back on the estrogens. "You seem to be flourishing on the diet," Sheldon said. "I wish you well."

I asked Sheldon if he thought the diet had anything to do with my recovery, and he said that he did not believe it did. "Maybe you're right about all the things you've been saying with regard to macrobiotics," Sheldon said. "We certainly don't have all the answers for cancer. However, until I see some data that support your arguments, I can't in any way support a dietary approach to cancer, or anything else for that matter. We may find in the future that nutrition plays some role in the cause and treatment of cancer, but right now I see no reason to start using diet as a treatment."

Nevertheless, Sheldon told me to continue doing what I had been doing and to keep in touch with him. He congratulated me once again and we parted.

When I left Sheldon's office, I walked over to Rittenhouse Square. The first signs of fall were in the trees. A new season was beginning.

The news of my x-rays hit the macrobiotic community as if I had been raised from the dead. There was a small party given for me. I celebrated by helping myself to some amasake, a sweet dessert made of brown rice, rice sweetener, called koji, and sea salt. Over the next few days, I received innumerable calls and messages of congratulations. Michio called me to offer his congratulations and asked to see me soon.

The reaction to my recovery at Methodist Hospital was one of disbelief. People had grown to accept the idea that I would soon be dead. The consensus at the hospital was that I had received a miracle. I wasn't arguing.

During the weeks that followed my x-rays, I walked around in a euphoric haze; I was elated, but shocked. I had been reborn on September 27. And like most infants, I didn't know quite what to do with this first flush of life. I had to restrain myself from gushing with joy at times when there was apparently no reason to be happy. I could be elated by an administrative problem or a huge pile of work on my desk. I began to appreciate subtleties of life that in the past I had neither the time nor the sensitivity to notice. I could hardly go near a bowl of rice or vegetables without feeling an immense gratitude to God. Insects in the air, the grass in Rittenhouse Square, the trees, cloudy days, sunny days, the great rush of life coming down South Broad Street—all of this and more filled me with excitement.

I didn't realize it then, but on the twenty-seventh of September I began an intense period of change, one that had been gestating since the day I buried my father, that day when I decided to pick up two hitchhikers on the highway going home.

Chapter 10

*B*EFORE I MET Sean McLean and Bill Bochbracher, I
had not read any of the scientific literature linking diet to
disease. I had read some of the books on macrobiotics, but
as a medical doctor I could not accept much of the
macrobiotic information. The macrobiotic view was not
put into terms that I could easily relate to. After the latest
bone scan, however, I felt a need to make sense of my
experience from a medical point of view. I wondered if
there was any scientific evidence supporting a causal or
therapeutic relationship between diet and cancer. As with
most physicians, my medical training did not include the
study of nutrition. I understood the need for certain
nutrients and the problems associated with nutrient
deficiencies, but I had little understanding of how the
overall diet promoted health or illness.

In October, I began to spend my off-hours in the medical
library reading the literature that examined the link between diet and disease. Of course, I had no delusions about
my own biases; I only wondered now if there was any
medical evidence to support my feelings. As it happened,

the studies linking diet to cancer were voluminous. When I happened on the scene, there were a number of reputable scientists who were saying that most cancer victims are done in by their own palates.

I began my reading with *Dietary Goals for the United States,* published in 1977 with a second edition in 1978. *Dietary Goals* was the culmination of nine years of hearings before the Senate Select Committee on Nutrition and Human Needs, chaired by Senator George S. McGovern (D–South Dakota). In the early years of the committee, the senators were concerned primarily with the problems of hunger. However, as they delved deeper into the issue of food and nutrition, they stumbled upon some startling information: an ever-increasing number of studies were showing that today's leading killer diseases were directly related to the typical American diet. Cancer was one of them.

At a press conference on January 14, 1977, Senator McGovern released *Dietary Goals for the United States* with this statement:

"The simple fact is that our diets have changed radically within the last fifty years, with great and often very harmful effects on our health...Too much fat, too much sugar, or salt, can be and are linked directly to heart disease, cancer, obesity, and stroke, among other killer diseases. In all, six of the ten leading causes of death in the United States have been linked to our diet."

McGovern made this rather unequivocal statement after listening to the testimony of some of the country's leading scientists; many of them were equally unambiguous. Dr. Ted Cooper, former assistant secretary of the Department of Health, Education and Welfare, told the committee:

"While scientists do not yet agree on the specific causal relationships, evidence is mounting and there appears to be general agreement that the kinds and amounts of food and beverages we consume and the style of living common in our generally affluent, sedentary society may be the major factors associated with the cause of cancer, cardiovascular disease, and other chronic illnesses."

Dr. Gio Gori, former deputy director of the National Cancer Institute, testified:

"The forms of cancer that appear to be dependent on nutrition as shown by epidemiological studies [comparisons of human populations] include: stomach, liver, breast, prostate, large intestine, small intestine, and colon."

Dr. Ernst L. Wynder, president and medical director of the American Health Foundation in New York, stated:

"Breast cancer, the biggest killer of all cancers in women, has a geographical distribution similar to that of colon cancer and is also associated worldwide with the consumption of a high-fat diet. Again, the disease is relatively rare in Japan, but increases among Japanese migrants to the United States. Like colon cancer, it is relatively uncommon among Puerto Ricans, who have a relatively low intake of cholesterol and fat in their diet."

Dr. Mark Hegsted of the Harvard School of Public Health, and later the director of the U.S. Department of Agriculture's Human Nutrition Center, wrote in the committee's report:

"I wish to stress that there is a great deal of evidence, and it continues to accumulate, which strongly implicates and, in some instances, proves that the major causes of death and disability in the United States are related to the diet we eat."

The scientists who testified before the McGovern Committee stressed prevention of cancer and other disease through proper diet. If Americans altered their dietary habits and lifestyles, they could reduce or virtually eliminate many common forms of cancer and heart disease, as well as other degenerative illnesses. The foods that present the greatest danger are those high in fat, cholesterol, salt, and refined sugar as well as those foods made up of refined grain products. Red meat and many dairy products contain large amounts of fat, while eggs and certain shellfish—such as shrimp—are high in cholesterol. Refined grains, which are stripped of the outer hull or bran, go into making white bread, rolls, and many other flour products. These flour products are also generally lower in other nutrients, which are removed during the refining process.

Dietary Goals outlined specific recommendations for cutting back or eliminating these foods, and thus reducing the risk of disease. The report urged Americans to eat more complex carbohydrates, found in whole grains, vegetables, and fruit; decrease consumption of foods high in fat, particularly saturated fat; eat fewer refined sugars and foods high in sugar; eat less animal fat, substituting lean meats, chicken, and fish; eat less butterfat, eggs, and other high-cholesterol sources; substitute low-fat and non-fat milk for whole milk (high in saturated fat), low-fat dairy products for high-fat dairy products; eat less salt; avoid overweight; and consume only as many calories as expended in energy; for those overweight, decrease calories and increase exercise. The report went on to make specific recommendations on how to reduce or eliminate these foods from the diet.

These recommendations were hardly popular with many industries—especially with the meat, egg, and dairy industries. Segments of the scientific community were also divided over the scientific justification for *Dietary Goals.* Yet, *Dietary Goals* started a landslide that was not going to be stopped. A year after the second edition was published, the Surgeon General published the *U.S. Surgeon General's Report on Health Promotion and Disease Prevention,* which urged Americans to adopt virtually the same recommendations made by the McGovern report. The Surgeon General went so far as to single out red meat as an important food to reduce in our diets, rather than simply saying we should eliminate fat and let the consumer figure out where the fat is located. (In 1980, the USDA and HEW jointly issued

Dietary Guidelines for Americans; these were basically the same guidelines as those of *Dietary Goals* and the Surgeon General's report, though slightly watered down.) These reports presented the U.S. Government's stand on diet and health, based on the available evidence. In light of the enormous pressure put on the bureaucracy by the food industry, these recommendations looked like the most courageous steps taken by federal officials since the Cuban Missile Crisis.

Never having read this material before, I was both excited and taken aback by it. The foundation was being laid for preventive medicine, a whole new approach to health care, and it was taking shape without any great interest being paid to it by a large part of the medical community. Since doctors don't receive much training in preventive medicine, or nutrition, they don't place much emphasis on it. They have come to see their role as one of crisis intervention rather than of encouraging the patient to take prudent steps to prevent illness in the first place. Thus, prevention flies in the face of a tradition as old as medicine itself: namely, that doctors work with the sick, not the healthy.

There are many other reasons why doctors have not stressed prevention. Science has been remarkably successful at finding cures for illness, and for this reason there has not been much emphasis, or research money, invested in preventive medicine. It is only because of the failure of science to find a cure for cancer and heart disease that prevention has been given any attention at all.

My personal interest in the subject drove me on. I read the studies supporting the notion of prevention with mounting excitement. Judging by the extensiveness of evidence, prevention is an approach long overdue.

In general, scientists have found four major elements of our diet that appear related to the cause of disease, particularly to cancer: an excess of fat, protein, and calories and a lack of fiber. As *Dietary Goals* and the Surgeon

General's report pointed out, the American diet is high in fat, protein, and calories, but low in fiber. It is also low in complex carbohydrates; most of our carbohydrates — which are converted into energy by the body — are derived from refined products, such as sugar and white flour.

However, this is not the diet that is common throughout the world. The typical American regimen springs from an affluence and agricultural abundance peculiar to the United States, Canada, and parts of Western Europe.

The diets of the East, in such places as Japan and China, and in the Third World, such as those in Africa and in the Middle East, are made up largely of grains, vegetables, and fruits. They are low in animal products, and thus also low in fat. At the same time, because these diets are high in vegetable foods, they are also high in fiber. Meat, dairy products, poultry, and eggs are all expensive foods, so consumption of them is limited among poor nations. (The obvious exception to this is Japan, which is an affluent nation, but has maintained many of its culinary traditions.)

Not only are the diets of the East and West different, but so are the disease patterns. Cardiovascular disease, cancer, diabetes, and obesity are epidemic in the United States, Canada, and Western Europe; however, such diseases are rare in many Third World and Eastern countries. It is only within this century that these illnesses have reached such magnitude in the West. At the same time, the quality of the American diet has also declined.

Researchers began experimenting with diet's possible link to cancer more than a half century ago, when Dr. A. F. Watson and Dr. Edward Mellerby found that if they fed rats high-fat diets and subjected them to tar treatments, the rats developed an increased incidence of tumors. In the 1940s, scientists discovered that mice fed a high-fat diet suffered more mammary tumors than mice on a low-fat diet.

Researchers then began to look closer at the disease patterns and the dietary habits of specific populations of people. In these surveys, known as epidemiological studies, groups of people with known high-fat diets were compared to those with diets low in fat, and then studied to see if there were major differences in the incidence of certain diseases. In 1966, Dr. A. J. Lea published a report that showed that leukemia and cancers of the breast, ovaries, and rectum in people over the age of fifty-five strongly correlated with the intake of diets high in fat. Following Lea's work, three international epidemiological studies were performed, each comparing the diets and disease rates of more than thirty countries. Overall, the researchers found that in countries where the people consumed foods high in fat, there was a consistently higher rate of cancer, particularly of the colon, prostate, and intestines. On the other hand, where the diet was low in fat, there was a low rate of cancer and cardiovascular disease.

Comparisons between Japanese health and longevity and those of countries in the West have also been revealing. Japan has long been highly industrialized and affluent. As a result, it has had to cope with problems similar to those in the United States: pollution and the associated health risks of sedentary lifestyles. In addition, far more Japanese men smoke cigarettes (60 to 85 percent) than do American men (43 percent). Yet, the Japanese show a very different pattern of disease from that of Western nations, particularly the United States. The Japanese have virtually no cancer of the breast, colon, or prostate. Also, heart and artery diseases are rare among Japanese.

One major difference between American and Japanese people is diet. The Japanese eat few animal products, and thus take in only small amounts of saturated fat. The Japanese subsist mainly on grains—namely, white rice—and vegetables. They have a high degree of salt, sugar, and chemicals in their food. Also, white rice is refined and lacks fiber and other important nutrients.

Scientists now believe that the Japanese diet—exceptionally low in fat—is the key factor in their ability to prevent certain diseases in their own nation. However, once they immigrate to the United States, they consume much higher levels of fat than they would have in their native country, and thus suffer from the same illnesses as Americans. The Japanese do suffer from a high rate of stomach cancer, and scientists have suggested that this may be due to the high consumption of salt and chemicals in their food.

The Japanese are not the only immigrants whose disease pattern changes once they settle in the United States. Scientists have found that Polish-Americans suffer much higher rates of breast, colon, and rectal cancers than their compatriots who remain in Poland. These researchers also reported higher rates of breast cancer among women coming to the United States from Ireland, Norway, Germany, and Italy than the national average for women who remained in their respective nations. In addition, cancers of the ovary and prostate increased dramatically among immigrants from Italy and Ireland.

Within the United States, eating patterns are fairly consistent, except for certain groups. One such exception is the Seventh-Day Adventists, many of whom follow a vegetarian regimen for religious reasons. This diet is much lower in fat than most American regimens. And, not surprisingly, studies have shown a much lower incidence of cancer, heart, and artery diseases among Seventh-Day Adventists than in the rest of the general population

Another interesting finding is that the incidence of cancer is quite different among income groups within the same country. For example, colon cancer is higher among the Colombian upper class than among the poor. At the same time, the upper-class Colombians consume a diet higher in fat, which would be expected because of their accessibility to expensive meats and dairy products This same trend exists among the people of Hong Kong, where colon and breast cancer are higher among the upper classes than among the poor. Again, the striking difference between the two groups is the level of fat in the diet.

How does this high-fat diet give rise to cancer? Scientists have advanced several theories, and most of them may prove to be correct, depending on the type of cancer. The most widely held theory is that fat appears to promote cancer by influencing the metabolic processes of normal cells, making them more susceptible to the development of malignancy brought on by other agents. In other words, a high-fat diet creates an internal environment that appears to make cells more vulnerable to carcinogens, which might not be effective otherwise, and it has been suggested that fat acts like a solvent, which enhances the effects of certain carcinogens.

Fat has also been shown to affect the metabolism of human tissue and throw off the balance of our hormones. An imbalance of hormones has been linked to certain cancers. The strongest case for this theory seems to rest with breast cancer. Fatty acids have been shown to adversely affect production of the hormone prolactin, which governs the growth and milk production of a woman's breasts. Prolactin influences the circulation of estrogens in the woman's body, as well. Abnormally high levels of prolactin have been found in women with breast tumors. Scientists have also found that rodents placed on high-fat diets consistently develop more mammary tumors than those on low-fat diets.

Not surprisingly, cancer isn't the only disease associated with a high-fat diet. Dietary fat has been shown to be a leading risk factor in the development of cardiovascular disease, including heart attack, hypertension, and stroke. Diets high in saturated fat and cholesterol tend to increase the blood cholesterol levels of humans and animals. Fat builds up within the walls of the artery, thus cutting back on the amount of blood that can flow to the heart and brain. Eventually, the condition, known as atherosclerosis, often leads to a heart attack or stroke.

Scientists have shown that a low-fat diet can reverse atherosclerosis in the coronary arteries of monkeys and the femoral arteries in humans. What effects a low-fat diet has on the coronary arteries in humans has not been demonstrated as yet. Based on the available information, however, there appear to be great possibilities for treating common forms of heart and artery disease with diet. At present, more than 800,000 Americans die as a result of atherosclerosis each year.

During World War II, foods high in fat, such as red meat, certain dairy products, and eggs, were rationed for the general population in Europe so that they could be given to soldiers. During the war and for some years afterward, the number of Europeans dying from coronary artery disease and heart attacks dropped dramatically. Autopsies done on European dead showed that their arteries were remarkably free of fat deposits. Many scientists today believe that this was due to the decline in fat intake during the war.

Fiber has been shown to be an important factor in preventing cancer, as well. Fiber, which is found in whole grains, vegetables, and fruit, is the undigestible portion of the food. Populations with high-fiber diets show a low incidence of colon cancer, diverticulosis, and other diseases of the digestive tract.

High-fiber diets have also been associated with more frequent defecation and more rapid intestinal transit time. It has been theorized that both of these factors are important in reducing intestinal disease, particularly cancer, because cancer-causing agents spend less time within the intestines and do not have a chance to accumulate there. Studies have shown that rats fed high amounts of fiber have fewer intestinal tumors than those fed a diet low in fiber. Interestingly, the observed number of tumors decreased in rats when fiber was added to the diet.

The structure of the gastrointestinal tract in humans is more similar to that of plant-eating animals than to that of meat eaters. Carnivores have much shorter intestinal tracts. This enables them to digest meat quickly, thus reducing or eliminating the negative side effects that may result from putrefaction in the intestines. The longer digestive tract of humans, however, may enhance the possibilities of this happening.

High-protein intake has also been associated with a greater incidence of cancer, particularly bladder cancer. Low-protein diets, on the other hand, have been associated with a decreased incidence of tumors and slowing of tumor growth.

Obesity, a disease that besets more than 35 million Americans, has been associated with a higher incidence of many diseases, especially cancer, and animal studies have shown that lean or underfed animals show a decreased incidence of tumors, as compared to normally fed animals.

The main controversy over these studies arises because absolute proof that diet causes cancer and heart disease is not in yet. No study done on human beings has convincingly pinpointed the mechanism by which diet might give rise to cancer, and as yet no double-blind study has been done on humans that shows conclusively that diet causes these illnesses. Without such proof, many scientists argue that public statements linking diet to cancer should not be made. They maintain that we should not extrapolate from animal data because animals may respond differently to diet and environment than people. What has been enough proof for one scientist is little more than coincidence to another.

Nevertheless, for many the available evidence linking diet to disease is formidable, and an increasing number of researchers and doctors have been moved to speak out in favor of prevention through better diet. Their statements have been controversial in themselves.

In response to this storm of words, Dr. Donald Fredrickson, director of the National Institutes of Health — this country's leading research institution — wrote in *Science* magazine:

"We've more or less become adjusted to the fact that we probably will never be able to get the ideal proof that we want...The weight of evidence seems strong enough so that we can direct people toward a set of guidelines."

And Harvard's Dr. Mark Hegsted wrote in his statement in *Dietary Goals:* "The risks associated with eating [the typical American diet] are demonstrably large. The question to be asked, therefore, is not why should we change our diet, but why not? What are the risks associated with eating less meat, less fat, less saturated fat, less cholesterol, less sugar, less salt, more fruits, vegetables, unsaturated fat and cereal products — especially whole grain cereals. There are none that can be identified and important benefits can be expected."

Prevention seemed all the more compelling to me in light of medicine's continuing failure to cure cancer. It was 1971 when Richard Nixon signed the "Conquest of Cancer Act." The "war on cancer" was launched; the act set 1976 as the target date for the elimination of cancer. This was to correspond with the nation's bicentennial, a point no one seemed to mention amid the festivities of the nation's 200th birthday. Since 1971, billions of dollars had been spent on finding the cure for cancer, with no demonstrable results.

Science has managed to extend the life expectancy of some cancer patients with surgery, chemotherapy, radiation, and cobalt treatments. Speaking as a former cancer patient, I can say that the quality of those extended years is nothing to brag about. The odds that any one patient will survive the disease are the same as they were in 1950: one in three.

More than a million Americans are under treatment for cancer in any given year, while each year 700,000 more are being diagnosed as having cancer. The death toll of this disease is 400,000 a year and climbing. Meanwhile, the annual costs of treating cancer exceed $20 billion. Cancer has turned into the most frustrating, costly, and intractable disease mankind has ever known.

With regard to the treatment of cancer, I did come across some information to suggest that diet could play a role. Good diet serves to strengthen the cancer patient and help combat the loss of appetite and muscle-wasting that is associated with the disease; it also tends to help the patient withstand the side effects of chemotherapy, which often results in diarrhea, nausea, and vomiting. Studies have shown that the cancer patient's life expectancy is increased and tumor incidence decreased with a diet that restricts calorie intake. The macrobiotic diet would certainly fit this definition.

In mid October, I wrote a paper reporting my own case history and reviewing the literature supporting the idea that diet is related to the cause of cancer, and then submitted it to several professional medical journals.

Reviewing the scientific literature and writing the paper served as a kind of catharsis for me. I purged myself of many of my own fears about macrobiotics and much of my residual skepticism. Intellectually, the macrobiotic approach made sense, especially from the standpoint of prevention. I still found it necessary to set the more mystical elements of macrobiotics aside for the time being. Until we had good scientific studies explaining how the diet works on disease from a Western, scientific point of view, I would have to reserve judgment on such matters. To some degree, I must accept the yin-yang dualities and ki forces as metaphorical terms, hoping that further research can fit them into a rational context that conforms to Western views of the universe. I could no more explain how such things work at this point than I could define how a piece of music can stir the soul. It has been my experience that the diet and philosophy seem to work, but exactly why they work will be left up to future scientific studies, which I myself hope to conduct.

Thus, the question of whether macrobiotics can cure cancer, or any other health problem, will remain a scientific mystery until studies exploring such a question can be completed. There is no doubt in my mind that the diet was instrumental in my own recovery. However, only through repeated clinical trials could we say whether the diet would work for others with different kinds of cancers, and under different circumstances from my own. I believe in my own case that the diet in some way triggered my immune system, which enabled my body to fight off the disease. This could very well have happened in conjunction with the treatment I received. Perhaps the orchiectomy in combination with the diet proved to be the deciding factor in my case. It is even conceivable that the estrogens played a role in the early going, perhaps buying me some time before the diet could begin to take effect. These questions are difficult to answer now. Nevertheless, there is no doubt in my mind that had I relied on just the orchiectomy and the estrogens, I would have been dead a long time ago.

Still, one case—or even the handful claimed by macrobiotic people—proves nothing scientifically. I am hoping that my case will inspire research that would show what diet's role in the treatment of cancer can be. In the meantime, the only prudent thing to do is to stress prevention through the macrobiotic diet, or one very similar to it.

For the next few days, I contemplated the possibilities of doing this research at Methodist Hospital. I also began considering the enormous potential in combining the preventive and therapeutic approaches of the East and West to form a truly holistic health-care system. This would require a new kind of physician, one who would be trained in conventional medicine as well as in preventive measures, such as nutrition and exercise. The physician would counsel his patients in preventing illness. Meanwhile, paramedicals would give classes in exercise and in cooking low-fat, low-sugar, high-complex-carbohydrate foods. The approach would require a partnership between the physician and the person receiving the counseling, since both would be deeply involved in preventing disease before it is manifested. The layperson would have more responsibility for his or her own health, recognizing that to a large extent one's health is in one's own hands. Of course, nothing will eliminate the importance of acute care, since prevention is unlikely to work in all cases, perhaps not even in most, since some people would be unwilling to make the necessary changes in their lives. There will, of course, still be accidents and illnesses that cannot be prevented, as well. This would require acute-care institutions, such as those we have today. Still, for people who want to make changes — a sizable portion of the population, in my view — doctors and health-care institutions would be there to help. This, of course, would have to be accompanied by a vigorous nutrition education campaign, alerting people to the dangers of an unhealthy diet.

Even in 1979, there were clear signs that this was the inevitable course medicine would take. Prevention means more than simply avoiding disease; it means improving the quality of one's life. Well before people have heart attacks, they often suffer from a number of other ailments — sometimes they are quickly fatigued, have hypertension, angina, heart palpitations. These problems debilitate them and reduce their overall productivity. By preventing the major illnesses, we are also reducing the stress of minor illnesses as well, thereby reducing health-care costs dramatically.

This consciousness has been spreading across the country, and there is every indication that it will continue to do so. People are concerned about their diets, their exercise patterns, and other activities that maintain health. Things are changing so rapidly today that what was faddist and weird a few years ago stands a good chance of becoming mainstream tomorrow. All of this swept me up into a great whirlwind of excitement, but eventually the tide of my euphoria began to go out. As it did, two thoughts became strikingly clear to me: I had caused my own cancer, and I had been given a second chance.

I lived the perfect formula for cancer: a high-fat diet, plenty of refined flour products, an insatiable sweet tooth, and a generally sedentary lifestyle. (I had only recently begun riding my bicycle when I fell in May 1978.) Little wonder I had suffered from intestinal disorders for twenty years. I should have taken this as a sign of my deteriorating health. My intestines were obviously having trouble digesting the food I was eating. Rather than change the food, I took medication to suppress the symptoms of the disease. I never addressed the underlying causes. Ultimately, those causes brought on my own cancer. Because I did not understand this, I viewed my lot as capricious and my cancer as outside of me. I had nothing to do with it—other than the fact that it had struck me down. It was all bad luck. My new awareness shattered my ignorance like a sledgehammer thrown through a window. I could no longer be so self-righteous or self-pitying.

I did not have any delusions that I had deserved a second chance, but I got one nonetheless. For this I felt tremendous gratitude, more than I had experienced in my life, and this demanded some focus. By late October, I started going back to the Roman Catholic church on an infrequent basis. I also started to pray daily. It was not in any formal way; nor was it charged with the sense of urgency and supplication with which I had prayed in the past. Then I prayed only in a crisis. Now, when I awoke in the morning, I felt the need to acknowledge my unity with all of life and the Creator, who set me on this path toward greater understanding and recovery. It was the opening of a dialogue. It was also the most sincere expression of faith I had made in as long as I could remember.

Chapter 11

A FEW WEEKS after I submitted my paper to the professional journals, it came back rejected. It was clear that my experience was not going to be embraced by the scientific press. Shortly thereafter, I heard from a writer who said he wanted to do a story about my recovery for the *East West Journal,* the macrobiotic magazine. The *East West Journal*'s circulation was relatively small—50,000 to 60,000—and most of its readers were either practicing macrobiotics or well aware of the diet and philosophy. I regarded the interview as somewhat in-house and agreed to do it. In November, the editors at the *Journal* informed me that the story would be published in the March 1980 issue.

Having done this, I began to speak out at various seminars and public gatherings organized by the East West Foundation on the relationship between diet and cancer. The main thrust of my discussions was that cancer could be prevented—and possibly cured—through proper diet. I also presented some of the scientific evidence to support the view of prevention.

In the middle of November, the New York City East West Foundation invited me to give a presentation in the city along with Michio Kushi. The foundation rented a large room at the United Nations, where a couple of hundred UN employees and local New York residents would hear us speak. I agreed to give the talk. Representatives of the New York foundation had agreed to meet me when I arrived in the city. I understood that we would have dinner together that Friday night and they would escort me to the UN the following day.

By now, I was increasingly feeling the need to wean myself from my dependence upon the Philadelphia macrobiotic community. I was finally well, and I thought it was time that I stopped relying on others to provide me with my meals. I was used to leading a life of independence, and I was not ready to give it up.

What made my dependence all the more difficult was that most of these people were so entirely different from me. Generally the macrobiotic people I knew were young, ranging in age from twenty to thirty-five years. A few were older and some, but very few, were in my own age group. I was approaching fifty. Thus, we were products of different historical periods.

Being a doctor meant something far different to my generation than it does to a twenty-year-old who is involved in an alternative health movement. To some macrobiotic people, I represented the institution most in need of change. One young man told me, "Doctors don't know anything about healing, but they know a lot about making money. They're real good at making money." One day I got a telephone call from a young person in Connecticut asking me to give a talk on how the medical profession was ripping off people. Another suggested that I had wasted the first fifty years of my life practicing medicine, and wasn't this regrettable. There were other such incidents.

To be fair to the macrobiotic people, however, it should be pointed out that this was not the predominant view, which is to bring about a marriage between Western and Eastern approaches to health and healing. Moreover, criticism of the medical community is hardly limited to one group today. I doubt that public opinion has ever been so ambivalent. At one extreme we have patients who still regard the doctor as the highest form of public servant; at the other are those who see us as a criminal elite, money hungry, and getting a certain sadistic pleasure out of putting people through torturous tests and therapies. In between the two are the majority of patients, who are increasingly skeptical of our motives, no longer fully trusting of our methods, but frustrated by the fact that they haven't got a better solution.

But this negative attitude toward medicine, where it existed among macrobiotic people, was not our only difference. There was also the problem of our differing lifestyles and attitudes. Many of the more mystical aspects of macrobiotics I simply brushed aside, but this was not always easy. One night while I was having dinner with the Waxmans and my regular dinner companions, the subject of Oriental astrology came up. Suddenly, everyone was analyzing personalities and events in terms of the Chinese Nine Star Key Astrology. I sat on the pillow on the floor and ate my meal and pretended not to notice the conversation.

Suddenly someone at the table asked me what year I was born.

"You've got to be kidding me?" I said.

"C'mon, Tony, what year were you born?"

"Nineteen thirty-one," I said reluctantly, between mouthfuls of dinner.

"Let's see, nineteen thirty-one. That makes you a six-white-star metal," Denny said.

"Is that so?" I said, still looking at my food.

At that point, Denny launched off into what a six-white-star metal sign meant. According to Oriental astrology, my nativity gave me all kinds of enviable characteristics: great ambition, self-confidence, strong will, leadership, stubbornness, tenacity; I was opinionated and possessed of a strong drive for spiritual pursuits.

"Oh, I see," I said, now finally putting down my chopsticks. "That means that everyone born in the year nineteen thirty-one has turned out to be a leader, an egomaniac, and all of us will die saints. Is that right? I seem to remember a few people in my high school graduating class who went from wood shop to the local jail, Denny."

Everyone laughed, but the subject of Oriental astrology often came up again. This and other mystical aspects of macrobiotics I simply dismissed out of hand. The fact that they were treated seriously tended to worry me, though, since it reduced the credibility of the information that otherwise seemed sound. I was constantly trying to sort out what I could make sense of and what I had to put aside.

Of course, I was not without my own faults. I often adjusted to new situations poorly. When it was cool in the houses during the winter, my first reaction was that the people were too cheap to pay for heating. I often reacted with a short temper and a good deal of impatience. Because I didn't understand the macrobiotic approach to healing, I was often confused and reacted to this by expressing criticism before all the facts were in, as in the case of my first kidney stone.

It is no small miracle that we managed to tolerate one another at times, and I thank God we did.

But as I rode the Metroliner to New York City for the talk at the United Nations, I began to realize how good it would be if I could begin cooking for myself. I really did need to get some distance from all of this; I needed a greater sense of independence.

I arrived in the city toward dinnertime. No one from the New York East West Foundation met me, so I proceeded to my hotel, where I awaited a telephone call. I had understood that I would be met for dinner. No phone call came.

Eventually, I left the hotel and had dinner alone at the East West, one of the vegetarian restaurants in the city. Back in my hotel room, I made a few telephone calls of my own, all of which proved fruitless, and finally I went to bed. The next morning I got up, packed my bags, and went down to the desk to pay my bill. Just then, into the hotel walked Shizuko Yamamoto, who had planned to be at the UN to hear Michio and me speak that afternoon. She had come by the hotel to visit me before I went over to the UN.

"Tony, what are you doing?" Shizuko asked me.

"I'm leaving. I assumed the meeting was canceled, since I haven't heard from anyone."

"My God," she said. "No one has called you. I can't believe it. Let me pay your bill."

It was not Shizuko's place to pay my bill, since she wasn't responsible for organizing the meeting in the first place. She insisted, however, telling me that she would get her money back from the foundation. Shizuko is a grand lady and took much of the wind out of my stormy mood. We then went out together for something to eat and then to the UN, where I gave my talk.

The New York foundation members all apologized effusively when I arrived, offering some lame excuses that they had gotten their signals crossed. After I finished my presentation, I got on the next Metroliner and returned to Philadelphia. As I rode on the train, I again considered the possibility that I might start cooking for myself. The only problem was that I didn't know the first thing about cooking. But I decided that over the next couple of weeks I would begin to take better notice of how the food was prepared. Meanwhile I would continue to consider the idea.

Ironically, while my relationships with many of the macrobiotic people began to weaken, my faith in the essential principles got stronger. I was convinced that macrobiotics would help everyone feel healthier and prevent and even cure many of our most intractable diseases.

In October, I began to formulate plans to establish a nutrition clinic at Methodist Hospital. I was fortunate to meet a fine young physician, Dr. Richard Donze, who was practicing macrobiotics himself and who was also looking for a way to incorporate this knowledge into his own medical practice. Soon, I brought Dr. Donze to Methodist Hospital and he began to run our small outpatient clinic, which provided nutrition counseling for those who wanted such an approach. At the same time, I had our cafeteria staff offer a macrobiotic meal to our employees as part of the lunch menu. It was not long before this entrée — brown rice and vegetables — became a very good seller.

The next step was to begin planning scientific studies on cancer patients using diet as a principal means of treatment. A couple of my colleagues expressed interest in working on such a project. We hoped to recruit volunteer cancer patients for the study. Our plans were to divide these people into four groups: those whose only therapy would be the normal medical treatment for the specific type of cancer; the second group would combine the medical therapy with the nutritional approach, much as I had done; the third group would be patients who had already had the medical treatment for their cancers without success and then turned to macrobiotics; the fourth group would be made up of patients using only the macrobiotic approach; these people would not have had any other treatment for their cancer. In any ideal setting, there would also be a fifth population, known as a control group, which would receive no treatment at all, but this would be obviously impossible to include. Still, some people cynically referred to the fourth test group, which would receive only the nutritional approach, as the control group, since the nutritional approach was the equivalent of giving no treatment. I did not share their point of view, of course.

After a specific time period we would review the data to evaluate the results of each form of treatment.

In order to do such a study testing the holistic approach, we would have to give up on the idea—at least initially—that we would find one element, or subgroup of elements, within the diet and philosophy that brought about the remission of the disease. Scientific studies tend to be geared toward isolating single elements that may bring about the observed phenomena. It is, essentially, the search for the magic bullet. However, if macrobiotics was going to be given its day in court, we'd have to test the overall hypothesis. This meant that the diet could not be separated from the philosophy of yin and yang, since the philosophy dictates how the diet is applied. For example, skin cancer—which is regarded as a yin form of cancer—is treated with a slightly different diet and external applications, quite unlike the treatment for, say, colon cancer, which is regarded as a more yang disease. Skin cancer is more yin because it manifests itself at the peripheries, or surface of the person, and is caused by more yin foods, such as sugar, fruit, chemicals, certain dairy products, and drugs. The treatment for this is a more yang diet. Colon cancer, on the other hand, is regarded as more yang, because it takes place deeper in the body and is caused by more yang foods, such as meat, hard cheeses, and salt. The treatment is a slightly more yin diet, composed of more lightly cooked vegetables and a slightly smaller quantity of grain.

I had some trepidation about beginning this study. Macrobiotics is the antithesis of everything Western, and my mind rebelled against using the scientific method to analyze it. The two approaches to health and healing point to the fundamental conflict between East and West. The Western mind is dominated by the rational-thinking, left hemisphere of the brain, while the Eastern mind is ruled largely by the holistic or intuitive right hemisphere.

Studies on the human brain have shown that the two hemispheres of the cerebral cortex are responsible for different mental and physical functions. In the left hemisphere, we find mankind's ability to think rationally and analytically. This part of our brain processes information sequentially. It is largely responsible for our ability to write, read, speak, and do arithmetic. It is also the left hemisphere of the brain that directs the actions of the right hand.

The right hemisphere appears largely responsible for the holistic, intuitive thinking in mankind. It is here that we are able to discern patterns, three-dimensional objects, and to recognize faces. The right hemisphere also controls the actions of the left hand and seems to be more proficient at geometry.

In *The Dragons of Eden: Speculations on the Evolution of Human Intelligence,* Carl Sagan suggests that the right side of the brain may well be responsible for manufacturing dreams. Sagan also points out that because such intellectual functions as speaking and writing are relatively recent in the development of human beings, the left hemisphere of the brain may have evolved after the right. He suggests that the left hemisphere could be something of a stepchild to the right, in that it developed in the way it did because it was not "fully competent" to do the intuitive thinking that the right hemisphere is capable of.

Dr. Robert Ornstein of the Langley Porter Neuro-psychiatric Institute in San Francisco offers an interesting theory on why the left hemisphere has dominated the Western mind. Ornstein speculates that the left hemisphere is exercised and its abilities valued far more in the West because of our dependence upon speaking, reading, and writing, and on logic. These abilities tend to obscure our awareness of our own intuitive abilities located in the right hemisphere, the way the daylight prevents us from seeing stars. However, as the mind begins to quiet itself, our intuitive and holistic abilities may become more evident, as they probably were in our ancestors, who relied more on intuition rather than logic for their understanding of the world.

Our rational, analytical view of the world makes us see phenomena quite differently from those who have holistic, intuitive understanding. In comparing the Western mind with that of the Chinese, the Swiss psychoanalyst Carl Jung wrote: "While the Western mind carefully sifts, weighs, selects, classifies, isolates, the Chinese picture of the moment encompasses everything down to the minutest nonsensical detail because all the ingredients make up the observed moment."

For this reason, Jung points out, the Chinese mind, which is dominated by the right hemisphere, does not separate the observer from the observed. The observer is part of the moment, and thus cannot be separated from any action that takes place within it. The Western observer, however, sees the event as preeminent, and therefore sees no relationship between himself and the observed event that takes place in any given moment in time. Thus, we see how the two hemispheres of the brain perceive life far differently from one another.

In treating my own cancer, I put this holistic view to the ultimate test and it saved my life. If not that, then it certainly was instrumental in extending my life and radically altering the quality of my remaining years. This experience was both exhilarating and shattering. I suddenly saw health and healing in a much broader context. This opened a whole new world for me. Awakening my own intuitive nature was very much like being removed from a long dark tunnel. I went from focusing my attention on viruses and cells under a microscope to sitting back and contemplating the vast interwoven mosaic of the universe. For example, when my back pain had returned after my trip to Florida in December 1978, I immediately believed the cancer had reawakened along my spinal column. The macrobiotic view was quite different, to say the least. According to Waxman, the origin of my back pain was stagnation in a meridian that ran along my back, preventing energy that had originated from celestial bodies and the earth from freely passing along this meridian and nourishing my body. The two points of view are good examples of Western and Eastern thinking. The former addressed the effects, while the latter attempted to understand the correct causes. Once I accepted the Eastern view as possible, I began to gain a new appreciation of the vast interconnectedness of the universe.

This is essentially the monistic view, that all of reality is part of a unified whole. The universe is one. As such, all of the parts of the whole are influenced by one another according to an orderly scheme. According to macrobiotic theory, the law governing this scheme is yin and yang, or expansion and contraction. Interestingly, when scientists look out to the farthest reaches of the universe, what they see dominating the interplay of matter and energy is this relationship of expansion and contraction. The same is true when we look deep into the structure of the atom. Beyond the world of particles lies this primordial relationship of expansion and contraction, or the attraction and repulsion of positive and negative charges.

This realization radically changed my perception of God, who suddenly became a far grander and more majestic figure than I had earlier perceived. It seemed, according to this view, that God had connected the most nonsensical detail with the most profound and far-reaching event in such a way that everything was moving according to an orderly pattern that mankind might learn to live with in harmony.

I felt a strong need to give expression to these feelings; I decided to turn back to my religious roots, which were the Catholic church. Yet, even though I went naturally back to the church every Sunday, I didn't know quite how the Mass and the church in general fit into my new spiritual view. On top of this, the Catholic church had undergone some radical changes since I last attended regularly. Vatican II had ushered in several major alterations, including the English-language mass and the playing of contemporary music and instruments during the ceremony. At first, I felt a bit awkward with these changes, but eventually I learned to live with them. I was still caught up with the form, because I had not recognized the union between my own spirituality and the spiritual essence of the Mass. I let it ride.

All of this in no way lessened my respect and commitment to science. I saw it simply as a natural complement to the holistic, intuitive nature of humankind. The challenge that lay before us at Methodist Hospital was to see if we could incorporate the Eastern and Western views in a scientific study. The possible benefits seemed enormous; I for one was certain that we could dramatically improve the usefulness of one approach with the other. Kipling was wrong, I believed: East and West could meet.

Throughout November and December, I continued eating my meals within the macrobiotic community, while my need for independence grew. At Christmas time I joined my mother once again in Florida, and for a while I cooked for myself. It turned out to be a wonderful trip and I thoroughly enjoyed cooking. I felt strong and self-reliant eating my own food, and decided then that I would begin cooking for myself when I returned to Philadelphia. In the early part of January, I did just that; I stopped eating my meals in the macrobiotic community and started preparing my own food. I was now Mr. Macrobiotic, as far as I was concerned. I figured I knew all I needed to know about the food and about the art of balance. After all, I had been to enough classes with Denny and other macrobiotic teachers. I decided that I could put together this alchemical mixture of yin and yang as well as anyone. There was one hitch: I tended to work long hours and there wasn't much time for cooking, so I decided to pressure-cook everything. Pressure-cooking brown rice is the accepted way to prepare the grain. This requires about fifty minutes; however, I found that I could pressure-cook all the other food in the meal in ten minutes. With two pressure cookers going on the same stove, I could knock out a meal in an hour. I would often cook enough brown rice to last me a couple of days. On the second night, I could produce a meal in fifteen minutes. It was a breeze, this macrobiotic cooking. After being dependent upon a small group of people for my meals, this new feeling of independence was just what I needed.

Meantime, I had become interested in Oriental diagnosis and wanted to learn more about it. In the middle of January, I called the East West Foundation in Boston and made arrangements to sit in on consultations given by Michio Kushi. One morning I flew to Boston and met Michio as he arrived at the Kushi Institute in Brookline to begin the day's counseling.

Michio, two of his students, and I sat behind a long, narrow table. Ten feet in front of the table was a large Oriental screen made of rice paper and wood that blocked off the consultation area from the rest of the room, thus affording those consulting some privacy from the many people who waited beyond the screen and outside in another room.

Michio wore his habitual dark blue, three-piece suit, white shirt, and silver-print tie. As usual, he smiled often and joked with everyone around him.

On that day — as on any other day when he did consultations, I was to learn — he saw the downtrodden and hopeless. These were the people who had tried everything else and were now at their wits' end. Many of them had cancer; others had heart disease, kidney ailments, multiple sclerosis; there were also those with domestic, mental, and spiritual problems of all sorts. Michio had a handshake, a warm smile, and a listening ear for everyone. Each person poured out his or her tale of woe. He let them go on until they were finished. Meanwhile, he watched their faces and expressions. Often, he would get out of his chair and examine the person more closely. Then he would resume his seat and make his recommendations.

Even with my limited understanding of diagnosis and of macrobiotics, I could see and understand many of their problems. Others baffled me completely. Yet, Michio never seemed to be at a loss, and after he explained the problem it all seemed rather simple. He had been doing this for more than twenty years and he had seen thousands of people; nothing seemed to strike him as out of the ordinary, and few conditions seemed beyond help. He would then try to inspire and encourage the person to make changes in his or her life. Not everyone could be helped, however. He often expressed his concern simply by saying, "It is very difficult. We won't know for a few months."

For most of the people, even those who had been told their conditions were terminal, he saw real hope and he attempted to infuse in them his own enthusiasm. Many went away seemingly determined to heal themselves.

Not everyone responded positively. Many were baffled with the macrobiotic advice and went away feeling bewildered and frightened, headed for what looked like an unhappy ending. Sickness turns many of us into wanderers.

For most he gave out the standard macrobiotic diet — 50 to 60 percent whole grains; 25 to 30 percent locally grown, cooked vegetables; 15 percent beans and sea vegetables; the rest condiments, soups, and in some cases, fish and fruit desserts, depending on the condition of the person.

The consultations ended after six. We were all hungry and tired; Michio hadn't eaten all day, save for a few toasted almonds that someone had brought him. I had to catch a flight back to Philadelphia and was in a hurry. Before Michio and I parted, I asked him, "Michio, is it all right to pressure-cook your food?"

"Sure. Sure. Pressure-cooking is all right," he said.

What I meant was, is it all right to pressure-cook *all* your food? He never understood my question.

I called a cab and just before I got in, we shook hands and he said, "Let's see each other soon." I told him I'd be in touch and then left. Little did I know what was ahead.

By February I was slowly becoming ill. I was increasingly uncomfortable and sluggish. By the middle of the month, I got the flu. Everyone else on the hospital staff seemed to have it as well, so I didn't think of my own illness as out of the ordinary.

I stayed out of work a few days, and then dragged myself through the rest of February. I was not getting any better, however. Meanwhile, I became increasingly intolerant of people. I became critical and at times outright hostile. I didn't know what was coming over me. I felt weak.

On March 1, 1980, the *East West Journal* published its story about my recovery from cancer. Within a week, I was deluged with mail and telephone calls from all over the country. It seemed that everyone in the country who either had cancer or knew of someone who had it—which amounts to virtually every U.S. citizen—had read the story and wanted more information. I later learned that people were Xeroxing the piece and sending it to friends and relatives.

Many of the letters and phone calls I received were from distraught people looking for any sign of hope. Initially, I took most of the long distance calls myself. I also tried to personally answer the mail. But soon both of these chores became impossible, at least if I were going to continue performing my duties at Methodist Hospital. Yet, the calls and letters continued to flow in.

I recognized a long time ago that I no longer just sympathize with cancer patients; I empathize. I know the pain and the torment and the hopelessness that cancer brings. I felt I had to do something to help them, if only to give moral support. Still, the litany of pain in those letters and telephone calls would have moved someone who hadn't been sick a day in his life. A mother asking for help for her son; a wife looking for something to save her husband; men trying to save themselves or their wives. Their numbers seemed endless. I had no easy answers. I wasn't even sure if what had worked for me would work for them. When the letters and telephone calls became too numerous for me and my staff to handle personally, I had to resort to form letters telling people to write the East West Foundation in Boston for more information about macrobiotics. Meanwhile, I continued to answer personally as many as I could. Soon, I was unable to do even that.

By mid-March, my health was rapidly deteriorating. I began experiencing hot flashes, cold sweats, rapid heartbeat, elevated blood pressure, and intense headaches. At first I believed the hot flashes and cold sweats were the result of having gone off the estrogens. The absence of the estrogens in my body, coupled with the fact that I no longer have testosterone in my system, resulted in the hot flashes. The hot flashes and occasional mild sweats had begun in June 1979, when I discarded the estrogens. Now, however, both the hot flashes and the sweats were worse than ever. On top of this, I quickly became feverish and weak. I couldn't deal with the pressure brought on by the *East West Journal* story. I had to get away.

I decided that I would fly to Key West for a long weekend and spend a few days on the beach. The sun would do me good, I thought. The following weekend I flew to Key West and took an efficiency apartment, in which I continued to do my own cooking. By now, however, I did not have much of an appetite. The illness did not leave me; I came back from Key West on a Sunday night in the middle of March with a sickly looking tan and feeling worse than ever.

Word got out into the macrobiotic community that I was sick and Michio called.

"How do you feel, Tony?" Michio asked me.

"Terrible. I've got hot flashes, fever, and cold sweats; I've got the flu and I'm weak. Do you think the cancer's coming back?"

"Don't worry," Michio said. "Everything will be fine. It sounds like you are too yang. Do you know Charles Hugus?"

"Yes, I used to eat with him at the Waxman house."

"Good. Well, I'm sending him down with my daughter, Lilly, and Josefina Gundin, our cook, to help you get well. Is that all right?"

"Yes. That will be fine. Thank you."

"Good. Good. Can they stay with you? If not, they can find somewhere else to stay in Philadelphia. It will be no problem. Really. What do you think?" Michio asked.

"They can stay with me. Send them down."

"Okay, fine. After a couple of weeks, let us get together. Okay?"

I told Michio I would see him soon and hung up. I was glad Charles Hugus was coming. Charles had left Philadelphia for Boston some months before, but while I ate at the Waxmans' house Charles and I had become good friends. We saw each other for lunch regularly, and Charles often provided me with macrobiotic counseling. I now looked forward to seeing him.

When Charles, Lilly, and Josefina arrived I was feeling worse than ever. The fever had persisted, as well as the symptoms of flu and the hot flashes. I was weak and generally overwrought. When the three of them walked in the door, my spirits were momentarily buoyed; the cavalry had finally arrived. They spent the next three days at my apartment ministering to me.

Lilly and Josefina immediately took up their stations in the kitchen. Lilly had the qualities of a Japanese doll; she had long black hair, delicate features, and seemed to smile a lot when she talked. Josefina was short, with an oval face and soft round features; she wore a kerchief over her hair and she seemed shy. Both women and Charles were in their late twenties. They settled in and kept the food and ginger compresses coming.

Meanwhile, Charles questioned me on how I was feeling and what I had been eating for the past few weeks. I told him and then mentioned that I had been pressure-cooking all of my food. I also informed him that I was sometimes freezing my food and reheating it later.

"You've been pressure-cooking all of your food, Tony?" Charles asked me in disbelief.

"That's right, Charles. Why?" I asked.

"How long have you been pressure-cooking all of your food?" he asked me.

"Since I started cooking for myself in January," I said.

"It's the pressure-cooking that's responsible for making you sick, Tony. Pressure-cooking all your food is like eating only one type of food, say brown rice, all the time."

Charles proceeded to tell me that pressure-cooking is a very yang preparation, which needs to be balanced by other types of cooking methods, such as steaming, boiling, and sautéing. By pressure-cooking all of my food, I had made my condition extremely tight and contracted, causing an extreme discharge, and my sickness. Charles pointed out that such an extreme discharge was very dangerous. In effect, I had made the same mistake that many people made in the 1960s, when they thought the macrobiotic diet was composed only of brown rice. Many people got sick on that all-brown-rice diet, and at least one person died.

Charles gave me massages and applied hot and cold compresses to me. Meanwhile, the fever and hot flashes began to have an impact on my mental state. I became increasingly hostile toward my guests and toward macrobiotics as a whole.

"If it had not been for the lousy macrobiotic community here, I would never have begun cooking for myself," I raged. "How did I ever get myself into this crazy lifestyle in the first place?"

I felt tremendous tension inside, and I was fast becoming hysterical. At times I lapsed into delirium and raged on and on about anything that came to mind. I also fell into deep depressions and succumbed to fits of weeping.

Meanwhile, Charles attended to me with the massages and compresses and the medicinal foods, made by Lilly and Josefina. After a time, my fever was reduced and my delirium passed. The symptoms became less intense, but I still felt weakened and ill. The hot flashes were also still with me.

I needed peace and quiet. After Charles, Lilly, and Josefina had been with me for a couple of days, a man claiming to be a friend of Charles's visited my apartment. The young man, whom I'll call Bob, said he was traveling, but to where and from where, I didn't know.

I would not have come in contact with Bob except that he insisted on talking to me. I was lying in bed and wasn't moving. Bob came into my bedroom and said he wanted to meet me; he said he read all about me in the *East West Journal*. He pulled up a chair and wanted to talk.

Bob found my illness amusing. As I lay there suffering with hot flashes and feeling rotten, he tried to engage me in a philosophical discussion, the topic of which was whether I had wasted my life as a doctor. Bob had a grudge against the medical profession, and he wanted me to admit that in my hour of need, the medical profession had utterly failed in its attempts to cure my cancer. At the same time, he also maintained that doctors were ripping people off. He wanted to know if I was ready to admit the futility of modern medicine, that it was essentially corrupt, that there was nothing superior to macrobiotics in treating illness and in saving souls.

I threw Bob out of my apartment.

A day later, my apartment seemed to be getting smaller and I wanted desperately to be alone. Charles, Lilly, and Josefina had already planned to leave, and I wanted them out. I was feeling much better for the treatment I had received, but I was far from well. The hot flashes and cold sweats still hit me periodically throughout the day, and I was still in the grip of the flu. In addition, I was still emotionally overwrought and the anger Bob had kindled in me was lingering. By midday I got out of bed and focused my animosity toward my predicament on Charles, Lilly, and Josefina as they gathered up their belongings and prepared to leave.

"Charles, I want you to know that I believe macrobiotics is nothing but unmitigated quackery, and as of today I'm severing my relationship with macrobiotics for good. I want you to go back to Boston, Charles, and tell your friends that. Good-by."

The three of them picked up their bags and went out the door.

"Good-by, Tony," was all Charles said. He then closed the door behind him and I was alone.

I got back into bed and went to sleep. Ironically, though I had lashed out against macrobiotics and my three guests, I never really doubted the effectiveness of the macrobiotic diet. My emotional outburst was the result of my hallucinatory state, coupled with the other symptoms of my sickness and my deep sense of fear and frustration. I found myself lashing out at life.

After I had been asleep for a few hours, I was wakened by the ringing of the telephone. It was a reporter for the *East West Journal,* who informed me that the *Saturday Evening Post* wanted to publish the *Journal*'s story on my recovery from cancer.

"No. I'm not going to allow another story written about me to be published. If the *Saturday Evening Post* publishes that story, I'll sue them. I mean that sincerely. I'll sue."

The reporter said all right and told me he'd inform the editors of the *Post*.

I got back in bed and felt death closing in on me. I slept restlessly that night. The next morning I got up and went into the kitchen. There was a considerable amount of prepared food left behind by Lilly and Josefina. Even though I had insulted my guests, and even criticized macrobiotics as charlatanism, I knew in my heart that I could never eat another way. I knew the diet was among the causes of my recovery, and I knew just as surely that if I ever gave up eating this way I would soon be dead. I looked at the food they had left behind; I'd be all right for a few days. I decided to go to Key West for the weekend. Easter was coming.

Chapter 12

I T WAS HOLY WEEK, during which time Christians mourn the death of Jesus and celebrate — on Easter Sunday — His resurrection. On Holy Thursday I sat alone in my apartment looking through the glass doors of my terrace out over Philadelphia. The city glistened like a jewel under the early afternoon sun. Inside my apartment, however, gloom seemed to prevent the light from entering, so that everything seemed cloaked in shadow. It had been nearly two years since I had had such an acute fear of death. It was hard for me to believe that so much had happened in those two years: all the surgery, the estrogens, the macrobiotic diet, the hope. Now the hope seemed all but gone, as I felt myself waiting once again on the doorstep of death.

Soon I could no longer bear the apartment; I went outside and walked a few blocks to a religious bookstore, where I browsed around for some spiritual literature that I hoped might guide me through these troubled waters. I found a couple of books, one of which was *In Search of the Beyond,* by Carlo Carreto, an Italian mystic priest. I had read some of Carreto's work before and liked what he had to say. As I went toward the cash register to pay for the books, I spotted a crucifix of the risen Christ, wearing flowing robes and coming off the cross. It was a beautiful work of art, a foot and a half tall, light and delicate, made of polished steel, with a wooden backing. The figure of Jesus was also of polished metal, finely cast. I bought the books and the crucifix and left the store feeling a bit lighter. As I walked down the street, I decided I would put the crucifix on the wall in my office.

For some reason I walked down Race Street toward Hahnemann Medical College, where I had studied medicine. It was about two in the afternoon; brilliant sunshine splashed against the trees along the sidewalk and the tall buildings of the Hahnemann complex. The first promises of spring were in the air. I had many good memories associated with this part of Philadelphia. Suddenly, as if I had mistakenly bumped into it, I came upon Sts. Peter and Paul Cathedral.

The cathedral is a mammoth structure—nearly the size of a city block—of Romanesque architecture, made of great dark brick, with a weathered green dome crowning its highest point. It sits on the intersection where Race Street and the Benjamin Franklin Parkway meet and form a triangle. Here, the cathedral waits for its flock, like some great ark ready to provide shelter against bad weather of all sorts.

Against the northern wall of the cathedral, at the Race Street side, is the chapel. Like a tugboat, it is simple and well used; most of the Masses are celebrated in the chapel, except for those on Holy Days, special events—such as a first communion, or confirmation—and the High Mass at eleven each Sunday morning, all of which are said in the cathedral.

I used to attend Mass here virtually every Sunday when I was a medical student. I remember praying for success in school—"God give me good grades" is what it amounted to. I was particularly devout during final exams. All I had to worry about was competition and passing tests. Actually, come to think of it, life had not changed much in the intervening years. It was still the big game of getting ahead, politicking one's way to the top. Ambition makes life complicated. For me, cancer made things simple again.

As I stood there on Race Street looking up at this grand edifice, I felt buoyed. This fine old church had seen me through some difficult times. Now I was troubled again.

I walked around to the front of the cathedral, went up the steps, and opened one of the tall double doors. The door closed behind me, and as it did, it shut off the brilliant spring day, with all its big-city tumult.

My eyes adjusted to the dimness and I walked through another set of double doors and into the cathedral. For a few moments I stood in the back of the church and gazed upon the immensity of the place. It gave the illusion of having magically captured infinite space within the confines of its walls and towering ceiling. The colors are what came at me first: old dark browns from the burnished pews and the marble floor; gold, from the gold leaf inlay of the ceiling; blues and reds from the stained glass windows. The lamps, which hung from chains in the ceiling, gave a soft, diffuse glow, so that one couldn't be sure exactly where all the light was coming from.

After my eye grew accustomed to the light and color, I could begin to take in the details: the long stretch of pews at both sides of the church; the towering marble columns that stood like soldiers to the left and right, separating the main church from the many smaller altars that stood in the shadows beyond the columns; above were the Roman arches, and above the arches were the stained glass windows, deeply blue and touched here and there with reds and whites. Straight ahead—far ahead from where I was standing, it seemed—was the altar, which stood under a delicate and ornate marble canopy that was supported by four more marble columns. The altar and canopy, replicas of those in St. Peter's in Rome, were in the center of the large, circular dais, where the Mass took place. High above the dais was the domed ceiling with its mural of the risen Jesus.

Against the back of the church, on the floor above where I was standing, was the mammoth organ; its many tall pipes all lined up looked like a mighty battery of cannons.

There was no one else in the cathedral but me.

The air was slightly scented, and my eye was occasionally tugged at here and there by the faint flicker of candlelight that gave off intimations of some mysterious life present.

There was no mistaking the feeling that there was some great presence here, the feeling that God was all about you, waiting for you, beckoning.

There was also a profound peace. I marveled at how set apart the world within this cathedral seemed from the rush of life outside its doors and walls. The feeling of a presence and of peace were so profound that they dominated the senses. No matter how dazzling and beautiful the church was, I could not dwell on it as a work of art. I was compelled to look inward, at the world within myself.

With my package under my arm, I walked up the main aisle and went to the altar railing. I knelt on the red velvet cushions and put my package down at my side. I prayed and my thoughts came quickly. My mind was suddenly clear and my memory all too vivid. I felt the weight of too many bad years on me. Soon I stopped thinking; I just felt. Emotions rolled over me like waves over soft sandstone, washing away so many outer layers until something deep and true— something even naive or perhaps innocent—came into focus. For the first time in a long, long time I felt love for myself and for others. Suddenly my chest filled with emotion and tears welled behind my eyes. I began to weep uncontrollably. After a time I collected myself and was exhausted. I felt enormously relieved.

I looked up at the altar and stared at it for a long moment.

"Take me back," I whispered.

I looked for a sign from heaven. None came. I continued praying and then finally got up and walked down the main aisle and into the lobby, or narthex. I opened one of the main doors to the cathedral and was immediately showered with light and the rush of life outside. Horns blasted, cars sped by me, people hurried down the streets. Philadelphia had not missed a beat. Again I marveled at the tranquillity within the cathedral.

On Good Friday, I boarded a jet bound for Key West. I thought another stay under the Florida sun would be enough to return me to health, but as soon as the plane touched down I became acutely ill. I got off the plane and was greeted with miserably cold and windy weather. I went immediately to the efficiency apartment at my hotel and got into bed. The next day I cooked a meal, but had little appetite. I was weak and feverish; the hot flashes continued, the headaches were torturous, the fear of death ever present. The following day, Easter Sunday, I barely made it to church, but the headache became so intense that I was forced to leave before the Mass was finished. That night I collected myself and got on a plane back to Philadelphia. I went to bed as soon as I got home, but I slept poorly. The sweats and hot flashes kept me up most of the night.

The next morning, I went to my office. My administrative assistant, Marie Genniro, took one look at me and said, "Doctor, you should see someone soon. You look ill." I agreed with Marie and went immediately to Sheldon Lisker's office.

Sheldon took me into his inner office and examined me. While he did, I had a full-blown attack of hot flashes, sweats, racing heartbeat, and elevated blood pressure.

"Tony, you're very sick," Sheldon said. "You've got a sub-acute case of thyroiditis. You've got to be hospitalized immediately."

"Okay, Shelly, I'll pack a bag and sign into Methodist tomorrow," I said.

"No," he said. "You're going to stay right here at Graduate Hospital, and you're going to be admitted today. This way I'll be able to keep a close watch over you." Sheldon is a senior attending physician at Graduate Hospital as well as a faculty member at the University of Pennsylvania Medical School.

"I can't do that, Sheldon," I said. "I can't eat the food you've got here." At Methodist I could at least get brown rice and vegetables.

"Tony, they'll make any kind of food you want at Graduate. Don't worry. I'll see to it."

I agreed and went home to pack a bag. I included *In Search of the Beyond* and some food that Lilly and Josefina had prepared, and returned to Graduate Hospital and checked in. I was given a private suite, and made very comfortable. Some preliminary tests were taken. I was sure this was it.

After a short time, the executive director of Graduate Hospital, Paul Schofield, came into my room with the hospital's therapeutic dietician. We greeted each other and he assured me that I would be out of there in a few days.

"Meanwhile, Tony, we hear you've got some pretty interesting eating habits and we want to be sure that you get the food you need," he said. "You should tell our dieticians what you need to eat and they'll make anything you want."

I thanked both of them and then asked if the food that I had brought could be heated and given to me. They said I would have it at my next meal. After they both left, I called Denny Waxman.

I told Denny that I was in Graduate Hospital and that I had been diagnosed as having thyroiditis. Denny immediately assured me not to worry about food while I was in the hospital. His wife Judy would cook for me and he would bring me food every day. I thanked him and hung up.

More tests were performed and they confirmed Sheldon's diagnosis. We are not sure what causes thyroiditis; it was presumed by my doctors that the flu had brought it on. In any event, the disease occurs when the thyroid gland, which is located in the front of the neck, at the base, produces inordinately large amounts of the hormone thyroxin, which causes elevated blood pressure and headaches. The thyroxin also causes the body to be hypermetabolic, which can bring on the sweats, hot flashes, hallucinations, and hysteria, all of which I had been experiencing. Sheldon came by and prescribed Inderal, for the thyroid, and cortisone for the headaches and swelling of the thyroid.

By now, because of the hypermetabolic state that I was in, I had lost more than twenty pounds and was down to 132. I looked emaciated and very much like a cancer patient. I was too weak to be overtly worried.

Later that day, the nurses brought a basket of fruit into my room. In macrobiotic parlance, I was in an extremely yang condition, and I craved fruit, which is yin. I literally could not stay away from the fruit. The bowl had to be continually refilled throughout the five days I was in the hospital.

Just after the nurse brought in the first basket of fruit, Michio called. He was lecturing in Montreal and had been told that I was sick and in the hospital.

"Tony, what's wrong?" Michio asked.

"I think I'm dying, Michio," I said. My voice was very hoarse from the illness. "The diagnosis is thyroiditis, but I'm worried that the cancer has come back."

"If you're still in the hospital when I've finished my lectures here, I'll fly down to see you. All right? Anyway, we should see each other soon, all right?"

"Yes, thank you. I don't think I'll be in the hospital long.

After I'm a little stronger, they're going to perform another bone scan. Do you think the cancer has come back, Michio?"

"I don't think so," he said. "I'll have to see you. I've talked to Denny, and, in the meantime, you should continue to eat the food he brings to you, okay? I'll see you soon. Okay?"

"Yes, thank you, Michio. Good-by."

After I had spent a couple of days in Graduate Hospital, the symptoms of the thyroiditis came under control. I began to feel much stronger. The night of my second day there Sheldon came into my room and said it would be wise if we did the bone scan. I agreed. I suspected that the thyroid disease was brought on by the cancer. The following morning I was wheeled to the radiology department and had the radioactive dye injected into my veins. Three hours later the bone scan was performed.

By now I was strong enough to be terrified. Graduate Hospital is a very modern facility and as soon as the bone scanner was turned on I could look up at the monitor and see an entire x-ray of my body. Thus, I could see how the dye reacted in my body, whether it had spread homogenously throughout my system or whether it clumped together in certain areas, indicating the presence of one or more tumors. I was afraid to look at the monitor, but I forced myself. What I saw brought tears of joy to my eyes. The dye had spread uniformly throughout my body. There were no aggregated areas where the dye might have collected around cancer cells. After the scan was completed, more x-rays were taken; there was no cancer anywhere in my body.

Except for the thyroiditis—which was gradually coming under control—I was well.

Once again Sheldon was in disbelief and, frankly, so was I. I had been given another chance. I was wheeled back into my room and was able to sit up in bed. After the nurse left me, I sifted through my bag, which was at the side of my bed, and pulled out my copy of *In Search of the Beyond*. I began reading.

"Let us keep this truth before us. You say you have no faith? Love—and faith will come. You say you are sad? Love—and joy will come. You say you are alone? Love—and you will break out of your solitude. You say you are in hell? Love—and you will find yourself in heaven. Heaven is love."

I put the book down in my lap and into the room walked Denny Waxman, his arms full of food, smiling in his friendly and somewhat apprehensive way.

"Denny, I just had the results of the bone scan and they're negative. I don't have cancer."

He was elated and together we could have cheered up the entire ward. After some short conversation, Denny said, "I've got news for you, too. I found a cook for you, someone who'll come to your apartment and cook your meals on a daily basis. You shouldn't be eating your own cooking."

Now I was even more elated. Having a cook would save my life.

"You're right, Denny. I can't cook. That's what got me into this mess. God, that's great news. Thank you. Denny, I'm eating a lot of fruit and taking these drugs. Do you think they'll cause any problems?"

"Don't worry," Denny said. "You're very yang. You got too yang. That's what made you sick in the first place."

Every day I was in the hospital, Denny brought food. I never touched a bit of hospital food while I was there, save for the fruit, which I ate with reckless abandon. While I was in the hospital, I reflected upon my relationship with the macrobiotic community.

Despite my hostility on several occasions and our differences over the previous two years, the macrobiotic people stuck by me. They believed entirely in what they were doing, that their efforts would result in the improvement of my health, and that my outbursts — when they occurred — were due more often to my illness than to my actual feelings. I felt a deep gratitude to the community, particularly to Michio Kushi and Denny and Judy Waxman.

Yet, I realized that there was also a fundamental difference between me and many of the macrobiotic leaders which represented the deeper, more fundamental conflict that exists between East and West. Our approaches to healing — indeed, to life — were so radically different that there was bound to be conflict at first. I had come to understand and respect — sometimes under duress, it seemed — many of the methods used in macrobiotics. It had not been easy for me, since apart from the problems that stemmed from my cancer were the obvious prejudices almost all Western physicians have toward the barefoot healer and the healing practices of the so-called underdeveloped world. Though they will rarely admit it, Western physicians must come down off a pretty high pedestal before they are willing even to consider the medicinal techniques of the traditional healer in Africa or the Far East. Were it not for my cancer, I would probably not have come down off my own pedestal; nor would I have deigned to consider the likes of macrobiotics as a treatment for anything, much less cancer. Many macrobiotic people whom I encountered had their own prejudices against Western medicine. Thus, my relationship with the macrobiotic community in general, and with some of its leaders in particular, was a stormy one.

Both sides had to deal with their shortcomings. In the end we had both changed enormously, and perhaps took the first steps toward a marriage between the healing practices of the East and West.

The day after I had the bone scan, Sheldon came by my room with his medical school students.

"Tony, I brought my students along to see you today,

hoping that you would feel strong enough to give us a little lecture on macrobiotics. I have informed them of your case, and the fact that you've now had two negative bone scans, and these students are very anxious to hear what you have to say. One of the reasons I'd like them to hear about your experience is because it doesn't conform to the textbook rules on how a cancer grows. And, as you and I both know, a doctor has to be ready to react to any kind of contingency, many of which don't conform to the textbook."

I could have embraced Sheldon. He was obviously doing this as much for me as he was for his students; I marveled at his openness. This moved me to forget the hoarseness of my voice and give an enthusiastic and animated lecture on the macrobiotic diet, balance of yin and yang, and motion of ki flow.

While I talked, I gauged the reaction I was getting from the students. From all appearances they didn't know what to make of me, and I had to laugh at the entire scene. Yet, after I had finished, they appeared interested and questioned me at length.

Word of my second bone scan spread through the hospital and for the next few days I entertained the questions of many of the hospital staff physicians who came by my room to ask me about macrobiotics. I was only too happy to give them the story.

I was discharged from Graduate around the middle of April and I spent the next few days sleeping and dealing with the depression brought on by the Inderal and the other drugs. Soon I regained my strength, however, and returned to work full-time.

One day shortly after I was back at work, I walked to the rectory of the Cathedral of Sts. Peter and Paul. It was a gray and blustery day toward the end of April. I was still hoarse from the thyroiditis. I rang the doorbell and it was answered by a young priest, who introduced himself as Father James Mateo. I shook his hand and told him my

name and then announced that I wanted to join the church.
"Fine," he said. "Where do you live?" Father Mateo asked
me this question because the church is divided into parishes
or neighborhoods. Each church services and is supported by
its own parish. One becomes a member of the church
located in the parish where one lives.

I told him my address.

"Oh, I'm sorry," said Father Mateo. "That's St. Patrick's
parish. You'll have to become a member there."

"Please," I said, my voice already strained from the
conversation. "I attended this church as a medical student, I
feel as if I grew up in it, and I want to die in it."

"Are you sick?" Father Mateo said. "You sound ill."

"I don't know. I had cancer, but I became well. I'm not
sure if it will come back, though."

"I see. Where have you been going to Mass?"

I explained that I had stopped going to church for the
past twenty years and had only recently begun to return.

"Well, I see no problem with your joining. Why don't
you fill out some forms here and we'll take care of you.
Also, you might like to consider taking our religious
instruction course. There have been a lot of changes in the
church since you left it and you might find the instruction
useful in understanding the Mass."

"I'd like that," I said. "I have one more request, though.
I'd like to go to confession."

"Fine," said Father Mateo. "Just follow me and we can sit
down in here." He led me to a small room where the two of
us sat. There I unburdened my soul. I described my many
years of selfishness, my overpowering drive for self-
gratification, and my unwillingness to see others as anything
but competitors. These were some of the fundamental
reasons I finally got cancer, I told him. I now wanted to
change my life. We talked for about an hour. When we
concluded our discussion, we shook hands and I left the
rectory and walked down Race Street to my car. The sky

was gray and unseasonably cool, almost fall-like; football weather, in the words of Fitzgerald. I felt as if I had just let go of an old and dying skin; I had just molted. I felt well in body and soul. Yet, I knew that if I was going to go on living, I would have to change myself fundamentally. I realized that in many ways I was no different from the way I was before I got cancer. I was still trapped in many of the same intellectual and emotional frameworks that I had been in before my disease, which to a large extent led up to it. The changes that I sought would take the rest of my life.

The following day was Friday. That morning, at about six-thirty, I left my house and drove to the cathedral for Mass at the chapel. It was a beautiful spring morning. The sun was just coming up; the sky was pink and turquoise in the east. The air was fresh and chilled, and as I rounded the corner and looked upon Rittenhouse Square, I noticed that the blossoms in the trees looked like tiny bells and lace.

The weekday morning Mass in the chapel is simple, yet elegant. The fact that it takes place in the chapel—a humble and almost austere setting—is even more appropriate.

Once the Mass began, I became lost in my thoughts. I prayed for guidance in a decision I had to make. If I allow the *Saturday Evening Post* to publish the story of my recovery, will I be providing false hope? I was sure that the macrobiotic diet—if properly used—could be beneficial to virtually everyone's health, and there was every indication from the data that such a diet might prevent cancer, and other diseases. But there were no data to suggest that the macrobiotic diet could *cure* cancer, even though I strongly believed that, in a large measure, the diet had been the reason for my recovery. And if it had done this for me, could it not be of great value to many cancer patients, as well as to many people with other diseases?

We still needed good scientific studies before it could be recommended as an accepted treatment in conjunction with traditional Western therapy. Yet, in the face of the enormous suffering that comes with cancer, the hopelessness, and the fact that we have had so little success in treating the disease, in light of my own experience with macrobiotics, I felt compelled to share my experience with others.

I have often wondered what my father's reaction to macrobiotics would have been. I believe he would have given it a chance. I'll never know. I only wish he had had the opportunity to make his own decision.

The Mass proceeded rapidly. Toward the end of the service, the priest prepared the bread and wine for the blessing. It is believed by Catholics that the priest has been invested with the authority to recreate the miracle of the Last Supper, when Jesus turned the bread and the wine into his own body and blood. Just before the congregation goes up to the altar to receive the bread and wine, the priest lifts the wafer high above his head and says, "Behold the Lamb of God, behold Him who takes away the sins of the world. Happy are those who are called to his supper."

At this point, the congregation chants the words, "Lord, I am not worthy to receive you, but only say the word and my soul shall be healed."

The priest then comes down from the altar and welcomes the congregation to partake in the Lord's meal.

I went up to the altar and knelt down. I continued to pray for God to give my life direction. The priest, Father Jim Mateo, handed out the wafer and finally got to me. "Tony, the Body of Christ," he said. "Amen," I replied. He then placed the wafer in my mouth; I said a prayer, and went back to my seat.

The message that came into my mind was clear: God has bestowed enormous blessings upon our food, giving it the power to heal.

When I left Mass that morning, I decided I would allow the *Saturday Evening Post* to publish the story.

I spent the next month recovering from thyroiditis.

Denny had made good on his promise to get me a cook. Diane Tredder, a woman who had been practicing macrobiotics for several years and who was an excellent cook, came to my house four days out of seven and prepared enough food for me for the entire week. Soon, my headaches, fever, hot flashes, and sweats passed and I was feeling well again. I was still taking the Inderal, cortisone, and an occasional Percodan tablet, but I knew that it wouldn't be long before I would be free of the medication.

In the beginning of June, I flew to Boston to see Michio. There was much I wanted to talk to him about, but most of all I wanted to apologize to him for my behavior toward his daughter Lilly, his future son-in-law, Charles, and Josefina. I also wanted to thank him for his support during a difficult time in my life.

We met in his library. His manner was as playful and comforting as ever, his eyes smiling. He acted as if nothing had ever happened, and when I offered my thanks and apologies, he simply brushed the whole affair aside. He wanted to talk about other things — my health, and the possibility that I might join him on his trip to Europe in the fall.

"Michio, I'm still taking a lot of drugs, the Inderal, cortisone, and sometimes the Percodan. Do you think they will cause any problems?"

He studied my face for a few moments and then gave me a quick examination. "No, I don't think so," he said. He advised me to gradually eliminate the medication and maintain a strict diet. "You need rest and you should eat very well," he said. "No oil, flour, or fruit. No fish. Eat very clean for a while so that the drugs can be discharged."

We spent the next hour talking about macrobiotics and the possibility that I would go with him to Europe in late October. I said that I liked the idea and would try to make the trip. He then asked me if I wouldn't attend the Amherst Program in August and give my talk on the scientific evidence linking diet and cancer. I said I would be happy to do that.

The summer proceeded rapidly. It was a time of recuperation and reflection. Soon, I was able to wean myself completely from the drugs I had been taking for the thyroiditis, and by August I was feeling well again.

In the middle of August, the *Saturday Evening Post* published the story of my recovery from cancer through macrobiotics. I had requested that the editors of the *Post* state at the bottom of the article that anyone wishing more information about macrobiotics or my own case should write the East West Foundation in Boston. I didn't want to be inundated with mail again as I had been after the *East West Journal* story came out. The *Post* complied with my request and it wasn't long before the foundation was deluged with mail in response to the story. Before the end of the year, the foundation would receive more than 35,000 letters in response to the *Post* article and the mail would still be coming in.

By the end of August, I was feeling fit and ready to go to Amherst to give my talk at the East West Foundation's program. The Amherst Program lasted a week and it was a busy time. There were several hundred people attending the program, many of whom had come after reading the *Post* story. My recovery also drew a good deal of attention from the press. I did an interview with the *New York Times* at Amherst, and later appeared on a couple of television shows. I was pleasantly surprised a month later when I read a cautious, though unbiased and open-minded, article in the *Times*.

On the last night of the program, Michio, Jean Kohler, two other medical doctors, and I were scheduled to give general talks about macrobiotics and cancer. The large auditorium on the campus was packed to capacity and there were many people standing in the back.

Shortly before we were scheduled to speak, Jean Kohler

arrived. I hadn't seen him in a year, since the previous Amherst Program. I was not prepared for what I saw when he walked up to greet me. One look at Kohler told me he was a very sick man. Gone was the healthy glow on his face. Now, he was a ghostly gray; his skin was so tight and drawn that he seemed to have aged nearly a decade since we had last met. His eyes had lost their sparkle and his manner seemed jumpy, nervous, and tense. Evidence of his effervescent spirit was still there. He was enthusiastic about being at Amherst and about the *Saturday Evening Post* story. His own book, *Healing Miracles Through Macrobiotics*, was doing well, he said, and his publisher had scheduled the book to be released in paperback. After a while, however, he admitted that he had not been feeling especially well of late, and he was still tired after having driven from Muncie, Indiana, with Mary Alice. I would later learn that he was still battling the flu, which he had not been able to shake since it struck him the previous March.

When Michio saw Kohler, he immediately expressed concern for his condition. He asked Jean to stay in Boston for a while before going back to Muncie so that he could be looked after by Michio and some other macrobiotic friends.

I was very moved by Jean Kohler's presentation that night, not for its content — his illness had caused his speech to ramble and jump around somewhat — but for his courage. He was obviously not feeling well, yet he did not let this deter him from the chance to inspire yet another audience to make a change in their lives that he believed would lead them to a more rewarding existence. He was a crusader down to his last breath. I didn't realize then how close he was to it.

After Jean had finished, I went to the podium and gave my presentation on the link between diet and cancer. I followed this with a short talk on my own experience, briefly outlining the facts of the previous two years. Then I got to the heart of my presentation. I said that I was the paragon cancer victim, not so much because of the specific details of my life, but because of the motives and attitudes that drove my life. I had lived a life of selfishness, greed, self-centered ambition, and fear. I was bent on satisfying my own appetites, and was intractable in my dealings with others. I viewed life as a dog-eat-dog existence; it was the contest of getting what one could for one's self, and the hell with the rest of the world. This kind of attitude made it necessary to be guarded in my interactions, and constantly on the alert against what I projected to be the selfish and hidden motives of others. Because I am an affluent American who, to some degree, has power and authority, I could easily satisfy my appetites. I had enough rope to hang myself. Yes, I believe diet was definitely the cause of my cancer, I said. But it was these underlying characteristics, which are so basic and so difficult to shed, that created the person who was attracted to such a regimen as mine and who ultimately became ill. This clutching for pleasures of the senses, and for material possessions, is what gives rise to cancer, I believe. And it is no wonder that the disease is epidemic in our modern society.

I told the Amherst audience that I do not know if what happened to me can work in any other particular cancer case. However, if there is a chance that this process of reversing cancer can be duplicated, I believe it will follow a pattern similar to my own. The first step in that process is to deeply reflect on one's own health habits and one's outlook on life. It took cancer and a death sentence to get me to reflect, and I can tell you that once you face your own imminent death, reflection comes easy. All you do all day is think about how and where you went wrong. One of the first things you realize when you have cancer is that you are not as rich or powerful as you thought. Cancer humiliates people before it kills them. This kind of reflection, of course, makes us see our priorities in a new light, and we are more willing to make changes if it means we have a chance to live longer, and in my own case a far more rewarding life.

The second and third steps that I took were to make a complete change in my dietary habits and to begin to pray, or meditate. By eating a healthful balanced diet, such as macrobiotics, I believe we can eliminate much of the disease in our society and a lot of the extreme behavior patterns in our lives. A simple diet makes us far more sensitive, if for no other reason than by eliminating so much of the fat that currently insulates us from outside stimuli. You can only gorge yourself on extravagant food—or any kind of extravagance, for that matter—for so long before you become insensitive to the world around you.

Once I regained some of my lost sensitivity, I felt the need to recognize my own dependence upon others and upon our Creator. As a result, I couldn't help but be more grateful for my food, the help others provided me, and the everyday experiences of life.

I have come to realize that everything is a gift—even our difficulties, which help us to reflect upon what it is in us that creates such situations in the first place. And it is this changing of ourselves, this spiritual renaissance, that is the path back to our Creator.

Once we start walking along this path, the first problem that will leave us will be cancer.

The following day the Amherst Program ended and I went to Spencer, Massachusetts, to spend a weekend at the Trappist Monastery before I returned to Philadelphia the following Monday.

At Methodist Hospital, I had several projects that excited me greatly. Dr. Rick Donze was still hard at work in our outpatient clinic, where he was dispensing nutritional advice along macrobiotic lines to anyone who wanted such information. And his practice was considerable. In order to expand his knowledge, Rick was regularly going to Boston to study with Michio Kushi. I was very happy with his work. To me, Rick Donze represented the new physician, one who combined the best of both Western and Eastern medicine to bring a truly holistic approach to health care. Meanwhile, our cafeteria was still serving brown rice and vegetables and the response by the hospital staff was overwhelmingly favorable. At the same time, a special committee of the hospital's medical staff was studying the proposal to do scientific studies using diet as one of the treatments for cancer.

Eventually, I took myself out of the planning of such studies because of my obvious biases, and the need to keep such a committee free of anyone who might have a prejudicial interest in the outcome of such a study. (At the time of this writing, the proposal is still in committee; however, the medical staff is generally in favor of moving ahead with plans to conduct such experiments. The studies are expected to get under way by late 1982, after the necessary funding is obtained.)

In the middle of September, everything seemed to be moving ahead beautifully. Then the wind changed. In the third week in September, I received a telephone call from Boston telling me Jean Kohler had died. He passed away on September 14, in Beth Israel Hospital in Boston, seven years after he had contracted pancreatic cancer. He was sixty-three. Dr. Michael Sobel, a surgeon at Beth Israel Hospital and the man who performed two major operations and the autopsy on Kohler, stated that he had died of an acute liver infection; his death had nothing to do with cancer, Sobel said. "For someone to have survived seven years with cancer of the pancreas without being treated is extremely rare, if not unheard of," Sobel was quoted as saying in the March 1981 issue of the *East West Journal.* "Something was controlling his disease." Kohler's autopsy revealed that his tumor, once described as the size of a fist, had now shrunk to microscopic proportions. These microscopic cancer cells were the last remaining evidence of the tumor originally found by doctors at Indiana Medical Center. Sobel said that the liver infection could have been brought about in any number of ways; it is possible that the infection originated from the exploratory surgery performed seven years before his death at Indiana Medical Center. Such infections often lie dormant for long periods before they become active.

The reason that the infection suddenly became acute is still a mystery. In March 1980 Jean had contracted the flu. In an effort to combat the illness, he changed his diet, according to Mary Alice. He never fully recovered.

The news that Jean Kohler had died hit me hard. Though we had had different types of cancer, Kohler and I were in very similar positions; both of us were battling a so-called incurable cancer with macrobiotics. The fact that he was still alive always provided me with hope and a sense that I was not alone in this struggle. Though there were others who claimed to have beaten cancer through macrobiotics, only Kohler and I had the kind of medical documentation that at least could be called "interesting" by Western physicians. Now I was alone in this fight. Then other things started to go wrong.

Shortly after I heard about Kohler's death, I received a hate letter from a physician in California. He had read the *Saturday Evening Post* article and was writing to say my remission was typical and had nothing to do with macrobiotics. My remission would not last for long, he maintained, and he hoped that the *Post* would have the guts to publish my obituary once I died of cancer, which would not be very far off. He was also letting me know that he was canceling his subscription to the *Post*.

I was stunned by the letter and immediately called Sheldon Lisker.

"Tony, all I can tell you is that your case is not typical," Sheldon said, "and that even if it was, I question the motives behind such a letter, since its intention seems to be to do harm, rather than good." Sheldon was very consoling. Fortunately, out of the many thousands of letters I received from doctors and laypeople as a result of the *East West Journal* and *Saturday Evening Post* stories, this was the only decidedly negative letter.

Nevertheless, the news of Jean Kohler's death combined with this letter shook my confidence. Was this doctor right? Would I be dead soon? What did Jean Kohler's death suggest about my own chances of surviving? The weight of these questions plunged me into despair.

By the end of September, the back pain returned.

It didn't take much for the fear of cancer and of death to emerge from the smoldering embers in my soul. When the pain first came back, I told myself that it was just my bladder meridian again. It would be all right. Soon it would pass. On several occasions, I applied a ginger compress, which managed to alleviate the pain considerably. I would watch how things progressed. Deep down, however, I was worried.

At the end of September, Michio asked me again to accompany him and Aveline to Europe, where there would be seminars given in several countries. I agreed to go. We planned to leave on October 17, and I scheduled a bone scan for October 9. I wanted to be certain about my condition before I left for Europe.

On October 9, I went upstairs to the radiology department, where Tony Renzi performed the same procedure that I had grown so used to by now. But just as I would never get over my fear of cancer, neither would I feel comfortable in the presence of the bone scan. The machine was for me a mechanized executioner. It was true that the disease did you in, but the bone scan seemed to announce the disease with a certain glee. Those wild clicks; those black patches on the oscilloscope: these were its laughing voice and hideous face.

As I lay there, I gathered my nerve and stared up at the drum, with its cross hairs aiming down at me. I forced myself to think of the trip to Europe.

Renzi turned the bone scan on and maneuvered it over my head. The clicking remained normal. I looked over at the oscilloscope and it showed no patches of radioactive dye. Normal. There was no tumor in my skull! He moved it over my right shoulder. Normal. There was no black patch in the oscilloscope and no change in the monotonous beat of the clicks. I began to breath a little easier. I told myself everything would be all right. Then Renzi moved the drum down over the area of my right rib cage and suddenly my every nerve was ringing with alarm! The clicking had shifted to an intense, rapid beat! My right side! Quickly I shifted my head and looked at the oscilloscope and to my horror saw a black patch in the monitor. Cancer!

Renzi moved the drum over my entire body; nowhere else did the bone scan discover any activity, except for that spot on my right rib. I was devastated.

I sat up on the table and felt the world go slightly out of focus; I looked at Tony Renzi, half expecting him to say something reassuring. He just looked back at me for an instant and then, with real concern showing, said, "Tony, have you gone off your diet?"

"No," I said. My chest felt heavy and I was suddenly out of breath. "Are you sure?" I asked. "Are you sure it's a lesion?"

"Yes, it's there," Tony Renzi said. "Are you sure you haven't been doing something that could have brought this on, Tony?" he asked me.

"I don't know, I don't know," I said. I got off the table and dressed. I went back to my office and made a few telephone calls. I tried to reach Michio but he was out. I left a message and asked that he return my call. Everyone I spoke to was shocked.

I knew this was it. My period of remission was over, I

thought. The timing was right. I had been off the estrogens for about sixteen months. My decline would now begin.

After I finished making a few more calls, I went home and contemplated my circumstances. I fell into a deep depression. I could not believe the diet had failed. I had widened my diet somewhat during the past few weeks, but not enough to bring about any negative side effects, I decided. No, the cancer was back, but it wasn't because I had changed my diet. Why, God? I kept asking. My one big hope was evaporating before me.

The phone rang and I picked it up.

"Hello, Tony, this is Michio. Is something wrong?"

"I had a bone scan today, Michio. I've got a lesion in my right eighth rib. The diet isn't working for me, Michio. I'm going to die."

"Have you been eating well?" Michio asked.

"Yes, I've been eating well. I've been sticking close to the diet. I've had a little binging, but no meat or sugar or anything like that," I said.

Michio issued a low *hmmmm* into the phone.

"Tony, don't worry. It's going to be all right."

Michio said that he believed it was not an incipient tumor, but my body's efforts to discharge the medication I had been taking over the summer. He reminded me that my condition was still delicate, and that any small variation, such as the heavy drug use during the summer months, would be enough to throw off my body's balance. However, because I had maintained the diet strictly over the following months, he believed that my condition would right itself with time. The food would see me through this discharge. The tumor would not spread, he said, but would eventually disappear if I continued to eat well. Give it a couple of months, Michio said.

Much as I admired Michio, I had a difficult time accepting so optimistic a prediction and thought he was just attempting to bolster my spirits. Besides, there was the problem of the back pain. I told him that though I realized I needed reassurance I didn't want to be deceived. Michio gave a small laugh and asked how I could still doubt him after all I had been through. He asked me again to give the discharge time and to continue to eat well; he said again the spot would eventually disappear. As for the back pain, he recommended I apply a ginger compress to my back each day; this would eliminate most if not all of the pain, he said.

I questioned him very closely and asked him if he was certain about this. He said he was. Once again, Michio said that he was opposed to my having bone scans, but if I needed that kind of reassurance I could take another test in a couple of months, at which time he predicted the spot would be gone. Again, he admonished me to eat very strictly—no flour, oil, fish, or fruit—for a while until I regained my health.

"What about the trip to Europe, Michio? Should I cancel?"

He thought for a moment and then said, "Tony, where will you work harder, do you think? If you stay in Philadelphia or if you come to Europe with me?"

"There's no question that if I stay in Philadelphia I'll work harder, Michio," I said.

"Then come to Europe with us and get some rest."

Suddenly, I believed him. He had been right about so many things before that my confidence in his judgment in such matters was enough to pull me out of my depression. If he says I can do it then I can, I told myself. I told him that I would go to Europe with him and that I would have a bone scan done before the end of the year.

The next day I took my x-rays to Sheldon Lisker. Sheldon was worried over the bone scan's results, but did not think I should resume the estrogens yet. "Let's just watch it a little while, Tony, and see how your condition changes."

I told Sheldon that I planned to go to Europe for three weeks, and he had no objections to this. I also said that I would have another bone scan in late December to see how the lesion was reacting. He agreed that this would be a prudent thing to do, and we decided to wait.

On October 17, I accompanied Michio, Aveline, and a couple of Michio's students to Rome. From Rome we went to Florence, where we spent several days. Michio lectured and gave consultations virtually every day. I gave my talk on the scientific link between diet and cancer, and spent the rest of the time touring Florence. From there we went to Paris, where the same routine was followed. The audiences we drew in France were enormous; most of the seminars were attended by more than a thousand people, some of them by more than fifteen hundred.

After more than a week in Paris, we went to Versailles and then on to Antwerp, where we continued getting large audiences. In Antwerp, I lectured to a group of medical doctors, many of whom were interested in nutrition as it relates to disease.

The three weeks went by quickly. While I was in Europe I managed to eat a fairly strict macrobiotic diet. I say "fairly" strict because I did two things which were not part of my practice at home: I ate bread almost every day for breakfast, and I went to bed a couple of nights on a full stomach. Both of these indiscretions were frowned upon. Despite the fact that the bread was unadulterated whole wheat, macrobiotic theory has it that flour produces mucus in the body, which prevents the system from discharging toxins as quickly. Going to bed with a full stomach is ill advised, because the body tends to heal itself at night, according to macrobiotics, and therefore shouldn't have to divert its energy to digesting food.

Nevertheless, when I sat down with Michio for a consultation before I returned to Philadelphia, he pronounced me well. He said that there were still some small traces of cancer within me, but these were in the process of being discharged from my body and generally I was well. I still had an infrequent back pain, which I expressed concern over. He told me the pain would eventually pass, and encouraged me once again to continue applying ginger compresses. He said the spot was not an incipient metastatic tumor, but a discharge of the medication I had taken last summer, as he had thought. I should not be worried.

On November 7, I went home to Philadelphia from London, while Michio and Aveline stayed behind awhile longer to visit the East West Center there.

When I got back to Philadelphia, I was feeling well, if a little tired, and ready to go back to work and wait for another bone scan. Throughout November and December, I managed to eat a strict diet. The cook that Denny had found for me, Diane Tredder, was just what I needed. Later Diane moved away from the area, but Elaine Rosner took over. Not only was Elaine an excellent macrobiotic cook, but she and her husband quickly became good friends to me. Now, when I attended professional luncheons or banquets, I had no trouble bringing my own food.

The fall soon turned into winter, as the city turned up its collar against the wind and snow. I had resumed my practice of attending mass each morning. I had still not worked out intellectually just how I should accept the tenets of the Catholic church, but the ritual of the mass was a way of expressing my faith in the wholeness of life, my gratitude for the gifts that had been given me; also, the mass became a source of strength and a comfort to me that I could not find in any other setting.

In the middle of December, I scheduled the bone scan for the twenty-ninth. I decided not to have the test done before Christmas because it would ruin my mother's holiday season, as well as my own. That year, my mother and I spent Christmas together with some friends in New Smyrna Beach, Florida. For those around me it was an anxious Christmas. I couldn't keep my mind off the bone scan, but I did my best not to show it. What would next Christmas be like? I wondered. Would I be alive?

I returned to a snow-covered Philadelphia on December 26. The wind came howling through the canyons of the skyscrapers, its icy teeth somehow always managing to bite into your neck. As I drove to my apartment, I felt vulnerable.

I got up at six the next morning and drove to church. The sun was not yet up, and its aura was just beginning to show over the buildings. I could see that it would be a cloudless day and that soon the sun would come careening off the snow to create a bright, almost blinding light.

One prays hard when one's life is on the line, and I was no different at Mass that day. I prayed that the lesion would be gone or diminished, as the macrobiotic people had told me it would be. If this did not come to pass, then I hoped God would give me the strength to face multiple lesions, and my own imminent death. As I prayed, I became increasingly afraid of what lay ahead, and like many desperate men, I was not above making deals with God, promising a new man should I be restored to health.

Afterward, I returned to my office and at nine went to radiology, where Tony Renzi injected the radioactive dye into my veins. I then went back to my office to wait the three hours before I would undergo the bone scan.

I knew this was the real test for whatever had been controlling my cancer. I had been off the estrogens for eighteen months now. If it had been the estrogens, in combination with the orchiectomy, that had been the sole cause of my cancer's remission, then it would make sense that the lesion would appear in October and there would now be multiple lesions throughout my body. We might surmise that the reason it took as long as it did to reappear was because the effect of the estrogens probably didn't wear off till September, when the back pain returned.

However, if the bone scan showed a reduction in activity in the right eighth rib, or even a complete remission of the disease, then I would have to conclude that the cancer was being kept in check by macrobiotics and my own faith, two things I regarded as synonymous.

The big question remained: Was this lesion in the right eighth rib a new metastatic tumor, or was it a discharge of the medication I had been taking in the summer, as Michio Kushi had said? The bone scan would clear up a lot of questions.

Just before noon, I went upstairs to radiology. As I climbed the single flight of stairs, I stopped at the landing, where a large window looked out over the snow-covered hospital parking lot. I looked out over the cars to some trees at the perimeter and then up at the sky. It was a high, cloudless sky of cold blue. The sun came in through the window and warmed my skin. I felt like lingering there forever. I prayed the bone scan would show a reduction of activity or a complete remission; to me the two would be equivalent, because a reduction would indicate that Michio was right and the lesion was disappearing.

"God, grant my request, I beg you," I whispered. I was so desperate that at that moment I would have promised the Lord anything in exchange for my life: I'd eat perfectly, I'd live an exemplary existence, I would be grateful for all of life. I searched the sky for a sign from God. The sky was silent. I turned away from the window and nearly knocked over a nurse on her way down the stairs.

"Sorry," I said, and proceeded up the flight of stairs and down to radiology. There I undressed and got into a hospital gown. I lay down on the table beneath the drum and waited for Tony Renzi to turn the bone scan on. I prayed silently and then suddenly heard the low, monotonous clicking sound; the dragon had been awakened in its lair. This was it.

Renzi maneuvered the drum over my head and the clicking picked up but remained normal. I looked over at the oscilloscope and saw the clear outline of my own head. Normal. Renzi moved the machine down over my left shoulder and I listened for the clicks. Normal. I checked the oscilloscope; it was clear. He moved the drum down to my left side and the clicking remained steady. The oscilloscope said normal. I knew where the drum was going next. I drew a deep breath and prayed. Slowly, ever so slowly, Renzi moved the drum laterally and held it over my sternum. Normal. The drum moved again, farther to the right. He held it over my right rib. I stopped breathing. For an instant, I went blank. And then I heard: normal. The clicking didn't change. I quickly checked the oscilloscope and gasped. Normal! By God, it's normal. My heart sang out! I could barely contain myself. Renzi very carefully maneuvered the drum over the other areas of my body and soon he had finished. I was nearly out of my mind with relief and joy.

"What do you think, Tony?" I asked Renzi.

"It looks good, Tony, it really does," he said happily. "We won't know for sure until I get the x-rays out and processed. I'll get back to you shortly, okay?"

"Okay," I said. "I'll wait for you in my office."

I dressed and waited for Renzi to come downstairs. The final verdict rested with what he saw in those x-rays that came out of the bone scan. The x-rays could show something that I could not hear in the clicking or did not see in the oscilloscope. Nevertheless, there were clearly no black patches and no intense clicking sound. I took this as a preliminary sign that I was indeed well. Before Renzi came downstairs, I closed my office door and could not stop the tears of joy from coming. I went to my desk and sat down and said a silent prayer of thanks. My entire soul was filled with happiness and relief.

Soon, Renzi came into my office with my x-rays. He sat down and told me that there had clearly been a reduction of activity in the right rib. "Tony, if you had just walked off the streets and had this bone scan, I would have to pronounce you perfectly normal. However, there is a faint gray area in the right rib area, and in light of your previous bone scan, this indicates to me that there is some slight activity there." Renzi told me that the activity had clearly diminished over the past two months, and it would appear that the lesion was disappearing.

"Whatever you're doing, Tony, keep doing it," said Tony Renzi.

That afternoon, I drove to the Cathedral of Sts. Peter and Paul. The sky was still cloudless and a far-away blue. The sun came down and ricocheted off the snow and ice and pierced the backs of my eyes. I was in the grip of a deep feeling of well-being, the likes of which I had never known. I parked the car near the cathedral, walked around to the front steps, and went in. The heavy, ornate door slowly sighed shut behind me, cutting off the brilliant sunlight and blaring tumult of the city. I stood for a moment in the semidarkness of the narthex, to allow my eyes to grow accustomed to the light. Then I entered the cathedral through the main doors, walked up the center aisle, and took a seat in a pew a few rows from the altar. There were a few people praying here and there, but because of the immensity of the cathedral, I had the impression that I was the only one there. I looked around and took in the silent splendor of the place. The lamps cast a soft, low light that reminded me of tarnished gold. The whole place was bathed in shadow and this old, golden light. Here and there a candlelight flickered, suggesting the hidden recesses of the cathedral. The silence and the mystery were almost tangible. Despite the immensity of the place, there was a kind of closed-in feeling about it, almost intimate.

So many months had passed since June 1978, so much had happened to me, and yet I had to wonder how much I had changed. Just an hour before, I was still grabbing for my life, seeking the attention of God for more gifts. I remembered a poem by the Indian poet Rabindranath Tagore, who wrote: "Time after time I came to your gate with raised hands asking for more yet more. You gave and gave, now in slow measure, now in sudden excess. I took some, and some things I let drop; some lay heavy on my hands; some I made into playthings and broke them when tired; till the wrecks and the hoard of gifts grew immense, hiding you, and the ceaseless expectations wore my heart out. Take, o take, has now become my cry. Shatter all from the beggar's bowl: put out this lamp of the importunate watcher; hold my hands, raise me from the stillgathering heap of your gifts into the bare infinity of your uncrowded presence."

My cancer was the result of my taking and taking until I had to ask for my very life. Selfishness is its own terminal illness.

Now, I wanted to live, and the only way to do that was to start giving. I could give for the rest of my life and not match all that had been given to me. Especially the gift of these past two years. That was the greatest gift of all — to be handed back my life and to be given this knowledge after I had squandered so much of my past. This was the lesson I had learned about true giving: that God bestows gifts even upon the unworthy. Such is the essence of love.

I would commit myself to giving the very gifts that had been given to me — to spreading this knowledge and holding as fast as I could to the simple virtues that lie within it. Therein lies the divine inspiration from which we could all draw strength and renewal.

I got up from the pew, took one more look at the altar, and bowed in thanksgiving. I turned and walked down the center aisle of the cathedral, passed through the double doors and into the darkness of the narthex. After a couple of steps in the darkness, I opened the main doors of the cathedral and walked into the brilliance of the afternoon light.

Mane Nobiscum Domine

Epilogue

On August 6, 1981, I underwent another bone scan at Methodist Hospital, the sixth test I had undergone in the past three years. The results of this latest bone scan revealed absolutely no sign of cancer in my body. The faint gray area in my right rib that was still in evidence on December 29, 1980, had completely disappeared. I have not resumed the estrogen therapy, even for a short period, since I quit the hormones in June 1979. The last medication I took for anything was the Inderal, cortisone, and Percodan which I took for the thyroiditis and stopped in June 1980. I was diagnosed by my physicians as in "complete remission."